Computer Supported Cooperative Work

Series Editor
Richard Harper
Cambridge, United Kingdom

The CSCW series examines the dynamic interface of human nature, culture, and technology. Technology to support groups, once largely confined to workplaces, today affects all aspects of life. Analyses of "Collaboration, Sociality, Computation, and the Web" draw on social, computer and information sciences, aesthetics, and values. Each volume in the series provides a perspective on current knowledge and discussion for one topic, in monographs, edited collections, and textbooks appropriate for those studying, designing, or engaging with sociotechnical systems and artifacts.

Titles published within the Computer Supported Cooperative Work series are included within Thomson Reuters' Book Citation Index.

More information about this series at http://www.springer.com/series/2861

Pernille Bjørn • Carsten Østerlund

Sociomaterial-Design

Bounding Technologies in Practice

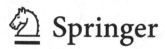
Springer

Pernille Bjørn
IT University of Copenhagen,
Technologies in Practice Research Group
Copenhagen, Denmark

Carsten Østerlund
Syracuse University,
School of Information Studies
Syracuse, NY, USA

ISSN 1431-1496
Computer Supported Cooperative Work
ISBN 978-3-319-38513-6   ISBN 978-3-319-12607-4 (eBook)
DOI 10.1007/978-3-319-12607-4

Springer Cham Heidelberg New York Dordrecht London

Printed on acid-free paper

Springer is part of Springer Science+Business Media (www.springer.com)

To Kasper
—Pernille

To my family
—Carsten

Acknowledgements

This book is the result of many discussions we have had since 2009, starting with Carsten's stay as a visiting faculty member at the IT-University of Copenhagen in the Technologies in Practice research group. Over time our ideas and writing continued to develop and expand. The book took its final shape during Pernille's sabbatical at the Department of Informatics at University of California, Irvine (UCI), in the academic year 2013–2014. During these many years, we have presented and discussed the ideas in several workshops, conferences, and seminars and many people have helped to sharpen the arguments. While we cannot mention all of those who have contributed to the theoretical development of *Sociomaterial-Design*, we would like to name a few who read earlier drafts and took the time and made the effort.

From the Technologies in Practice research group at the IT University of Copenhagen, we would like to mention Nina Boulus-Rødje, Casper Bruun Jensen, Laura Watts, and Debra Howcroft, who read early drafts of chapters and spent time providing us with feedback that helped to create our argument. Also we would like to mention Pernille's current and former PhD students Naja Holten Møller and Stina Matthiesen, and in particular Rasmus Eskild Jensen who read an early complete version of the book.

From the Department of Informatics, UCI, we would like to acknowledge Melissa Mazmania and Katie Pine who provided feedback on some of the early chapters, and Paul Dourish and his group of PhD students and postdocs affiliated with the Intel ISTC centre, including: Silvia Lindtner, Morgan Ames, Marisa Cohn, and Lilly Nguyen, for their supportive engagement. We would also like to acknowledge other great people from UCI, who contributed directly to this book in diverse ways, including Geof Bowker for his engagement in discussing different publishing approaches for this book; Yunan Chen and her students for providing the opportunity to discuss the book content related to healthcare research and technology design; and Martha Feldman and her practice theory reading group who volunteered to read parts of the book, providing the opportunity to discuss the content related to practice theory and sociomateriality.

Finally, we would like to mention Bonnie Nardi, who read an early version of the complete manuscript and provided feedback, as well as Wanda Orlikowski who took the time to provide us with overall comments and support for our project.

Thank you to all. We appreciate your discussions and time.

2014   Pernille Bjørn
                                                          & Carsten Østerlund

Contents

Chapter 1
Introduction

1.1 Story of a Sociomaterial-Designer

A sociomaterial-designer walks into an emergency department (ED). It is a very busy environment where nurses, doctors, paramedics, patients, clerks, cleaners, and others are moving around exchanging documents, clipboards, test results, and fluid samples while annotating coordinative artefacts such as whiteboards or paper forms. At first, when the sociomaterial-designer arrives, she feels overwhelmed by what she sees. The sociomaterial practices appear complex, dynamic, and highly entangled, and individual activities—such as the arrival of a patient who requires immediate resuscitation—send ripples through the whole ED. Such activities involve not only the healthcare practitioners attending to the new patient, but also the dynamic state of the sociomaterial practices that make up the ED.

The sociomaterial-designer enters the ED for a reason. She has an aim and an interest: Namely to design a digital whiteboard that can replace the existing dry erase whiteboard. The new whiteboard's purpose is to create new improved conditions for ED staff as they coordinate in a team effort when receiving and stabilizing patients before they are assigned to a ward in the hospital, an out-patient clinic, or are sent home. The sociomaterial-designer knows that the physical properties of coordinative artefacts matter by conditioning in particular ways, in which sociomaterial practices can occur. Therefore, the sociomaterial-designer must carefully consider how the creation of new technological innovations such as coordinative artefacts should be made and out of which material properties.

The sociomaterial-designer can design an artefact, but cannot design sociomaterial practices. Sociomaterial practices emerge in practice and, therefore, cannot be designed. However, the design of artefacts will condition the sociomaterial space for interaction, since when enacted in practice, the artefact becomes part of what constitutes the sociomaterial practice. Not knowing what the future sociomaterial practices will look like, the sociomaterial-designer will begin the design practice by paying attention to what is available visibly, namely the current sociomaterial

© Springer International Publishing Switzerland 2014

P. Bjørn, C. Østerlund, *Sociomaterial-Design*, Computer Supported Cooperative Work,
DOI 10.1007/978-3-319-12607-4_1

practices of existing artefacts. In our example, the designer starts by zooming in on the dry erase whiteboards in the back end of the ED. There are two whiteboards: One at the "fast track" side and one at the "acute" side. Fast track patients leave the ED fast since their conditions do not require long term monitoring and treatment, while acute patients typically stay longer in the ED. These two whiteboards have different material properties and are enacted in different ways. The sociomaterial-designer begins by focusing on the whiteboard at the acute side of the ED.

At first, the whiteboard appears as a single object, approximately 2 m long and 1 m tall. There is a permanent table structure that has been drawn on the white-board on which the column furthest to the left is labeled "Locations" and below is a list of all the locations available for patients in the ED (like cubicle numbers, as well as special rooms such as the suture room). While the specific locations are permanently drawn on the whiteboard, the rest of the whiteboard only contains permanent labels at the top of the columns, but the space below is used for filling in information with erasable markers. The sociomaterial-designer pays attention to the current whiteboard as a singular artefact and, at first, observes all the different annotation and practices for filling in the whiteboard. However, she is aware that the boundaries making the whiteboard cannot simply be detected by focusing on the whiteboard only as a singular artefact. Rather artefacts are sociomaterial enti-ties, which means that they "come to life" through enactments in practice also refer to as *boundings*. Sociomaterial boundings are the practices that *bind-together* in a hyphened structure while creating the boundaries for what is inside and what is outside, as in [bracketing-structures], of the sociomaterial artefact. The question be-comes: What makes the boundaries for the whiteboard as a sociomaterial artefact? Further, how are the sociomaterial boundaries for the whiteboard enacted? What is the space for design?

The sociomaterial-designer recognizes that countless bounding practices are part of what make the whiteboard constitutive of the sociomaterial practices within the ED. Thus, the question is about which boundings the sociomaterial-designer should pay attention to, since it would be futile to consider them all. Mainly, three types of boundings are important when we explore the sociomaterial practices of coordina-tive artefacts: The bounding of multiple artefacts, the bounding of artefact and loca-tion, and the bounding of artefact and people's movements. Each bounding does not tell the full story, but together these provide three agential cuts into reality that are critical when designing coordinative artefacts.

Exploring the three boundings, new and important insights into the space for design emerge. Firstly, by paying attention to how the whiteboard is *bounded with other artefacts*, the connections between the chart rack below the whiteboard and, thus, with all the clipboards (each representing all patients current present in the ED) become visible. To understand the sociomaterial practices, which emerge through the enactment of the artefact, it is critical to take note of what makes the boundar-ies for the artefact as a multiplicity. Exploring the bounding of the whiteboard as a multiplicity the whiteboard emerges as: [whiteboard-chart-rack-clipboard-patient-in-room-3-having-IV]. The whiteboard becomes bounded within the sociomaterial practices, through the practices where nurses and doctors connect and relate the whiteboard to the clipboard, the chart rack, and to the particular patient located in a particular room at a particular time. Boundings are temporal in nature and constantly changing as practices emerge. These sociomaterial relations must be considered for the design of the digital whiteboard and, as such, when designing the material properties of the whiteboard. The sociomaterial-designer knows that it is crucial for new digital artefacts not to disconnect important relations. Or at the very least, the design of new digital artefacts should consider how disconnected relations could be re-configured to ensure supportive work environment conditions for the healthcare professional.

Secondly, the sociomaterial-designer attends to how the whiteboard is *bounded with locations*. Here it becomes visible that the sociomaterial connections in which the whiteboard is enacted include the bounding between the artefact and diverse locations. "Location" is a column pre-drawn on the whiteboard on the acute side of the receiving area, because acute patients are not moved between cubicles. Zooming in a little more on the details on the acute whiteboard we find that part of what *makes* a "location" in the ED is the state of the location, such as the state of the cubicle. The state of a cubicle is a categorization scheme where the location can be "clean," "full," "dirty," and "terminal clean." When a location is clean, it is possible for nurses to allocate the space for a new patient, but in the three other cases the room is not available. Either a patient occupies the cubicle or the patient has left the cubicle, which then needs to be cleaned by housekeeping. This observation brings our attention to the work that is often neglected when we design electronic systems, namely lower-status work such as housekeeping. While nurses and physicians are invited into the design process in most cases, rarely do we find secretaries or housekeepers involved. While housekeeping seldom is included within the design of digital systems in healthcare, our sociomaterial-designer pays attention to the critical part of housekeeping as it is part of what constitutes the work in the ED. Zooming in on housekeeping's use of the whiteboard, it becomes clear that the cleaning personnel make particular annotations to indicate the state of the locations. For example, terminal clean entails that housekeeping staff have to clean everything in the room (including walls), and afterwards the room has to be left unoccupied for a period of time (almost an hour) to ensure that the former patient with an infectious disease does not spread the disease to other patients. This entails that the housekeeping staff have different types of annotation categories used directly on the whiteboard to indicate the type of cleaning. When focusing on location, the bounding practices of the whiteboard thus emerge as the multiplicity of [whiteboard-housekeeping-locations-state-of-location-time-before-new-patients-can-arrive]. What we see here is that the bounding between artefact and location renders the artefact a new type of multiplicity different from, for example, the bounding of multiple artefacts, and thus sets new conditions for the space for design. How will the new design of the whiteboard take into account the important connections between, for instance, locations and housekeeping?

The final bounding that the sociomaterial-designer considers is how the whiteboard is *bounded with people's movements*. Emergency employees move a lot, and what makes up one of the critical connections between the whiteboard and how people move are the sociomaterial-practices involved in coordinating nurses' breaks. Nurses work in 12 h shifts, and there are always between seven and ten nurses present in the ED around the clock, seven days a week, year-round. Due to nurses' long working hours, it is critical that they get breaks during their shifts to ensure quality work. When the sociomaterial-designer explores nursing breaks, it quickly becomes evident that there is a practice of writing the names of nurses on duty on the whiteboard, each with a designated number indicating in which order they can take their breaks. This system takes into account the nurses' individual training, such as variables like which nurses are qualified to take on the responsibility of triage. Nurses' names are also written on the whiteboard next to the rows listing the patients they are responsible for. Each time a nurse goes on break, following the ordered listed at the top of the whiteboard, it has ripple effects on the whole whiteboard. The nurse will be responsible for one to several patients, and for each patient she will have her name written in the patient row under the column "nurse." When she leaves for her break, her name is replaced by the name of the nurse who will take charge of that patient (the "break nurse") while she is away. Thus, the name of the "break nurse" will replace the name of the nurse on-duty in the column "nurse." Nurses move around the ED assuming different roles at different times (triage nurse, fast track nurse, chart nurse, break nurse, etc.). The nursing categories all give indication of location and movement beside skills and competences. Thus, focusing on the bounding of the whiteboard and movement, the multiplicity that arises comprises [whiteboard-nursing-breaks-nurse-role-break-order-fast-track-location-triage-desk-location].

These three types of boundings each allow the sociomaterial-designer to explore the sociomaterial practices upon which the whiteboard is enacted. The whiteboard emerges as a multiplicities dynamically changing over temporal events and patterns. Each bounding creates different boundaries for what makes the artefact at particular times. Each *bounding* is thus a temporal and dynamic practice by which artefacts are enacted, through binding together artefacts, location, and movement in diverse ways while setting the boundaries for what is inside or outside the sociomaterial entity at different points in time. Each bounding is relevant when deciding the design space for digital artefacts. It is important to keep in mind that all boundings are temporal and dynamic, which means they are constantly changing. The boundings can only be stabilized and observed by stopping the clock and examining what makes the boundaries for the artefact within a particular timeframe. In addition, the sociomaterial-designer has to take into account how the different types of whiteboards that are all part of the ED have come into being and practice. For example, the whiteboard at fast track is enacted quite differently from the whiteboard at the acute side, and the sociomaterial-designer described in this narrative has not yet unpacked these practices. When the sociomaterial-designer leaves the ED and enters into the design lab, the space for design is set by the insights into the different types of bounding. It could be that designing the digital whiteboard is not about designing a large screen with the same permanent table structure, but instead about designing an artefact with flexible boundaries. It could also be that, at times, what constitutes the whiteboard are the movements of housekeeping personnel and their annotations of the state of the rooms, entered through connected devices on the walls of the cubicles. Then, at other times, what makes the boundaries of the whiteboard could include the location of the nurses; for instance, are they at the triage desk or in the suture room? This could indicate that the whiteboard serves many more purposes and roles than what can be designed for a digital screen at the nurses' station. Digital whiteboards in the ED may have to be part of a collaborative system designed to support the work of healthcare professionals dispersed in various locations and enacting different boundings. What becomes included in the sociomaterial practices when dynamic artefacts are enacted? When coordinative artefacts are designed they can sometimes be bendable, soft, yellow, or transparent depending upon the bounding practices that define the artefact. Therefore, the sociomaterial-designer needs a tool or an instrument to explore the current sociomaterial practices, with the aim of identifying the space for design of the material matter of the artefact. The sociomaterial-designer insists that matter matters, but that we can only understand how it matters when examining the artefacts in practice. The larger design question is: How can we design an artefact without pre-determined boundaries? How can we design an artefact that is malleable and dynamic while still remaining the same? These are the questions that this book will explore.

1.2 Why Sociomaterial-Design?

Research on human agency and information technology is an interdisciplinary inquiry, which is explored in a range of fields such as informatics, communications, computer-human interaction (CHI), information systems (IS), computer-supported cooperative work (CSCW), participatory design (PC), as well as philosophy, science, and technology studies (STS) (e.g. Bødker 1991; Bowker and Star 2002; Schmidt 2011; Simonsen and Robertsen 2013). The common interest is to explore the basic nature of work, collaboration, organization, technologies, and human agency, and how such understandings, vocabularies, and conceptualizations can create active interventions in the design and construction processes of technologies. Another shared interest is in helping to understand how technologies are made and enacted in practices. Working in interdisciplinary research environments one is often questioned on the very foundation of the research one does, and how this research together with other disciplinary approaches can help illuminate a common problem or complexity encountered in the world. Several prominent researchers (Berg 1997; Dourish 2004; Suchman 2007) take these opportunities for interaction between fields seriously and dive into the very core of such questions, unpacking the interdisciplinary nature of common interests. This book has as its core mission to unite these initiatives and dive into the interdisciplinary, revealing the intersections between two seemingly contrasting research interests—*sociomateriality* and *design*—and in bridging them, create something new—*sociomaterial-design*. But why is sociomaterial-design important and why is it needed now?

The emerging literature on sociomateriality (e.g. Orlikowski 2007; Leonardi et al. 2012; Jones 2013) offers an epistemological and ontological foundation for articulating the intra-actions among heterogeneous actors, artefacts, and activities (Law 2004; Suchman 2007). A sociomaterial perspective allows us to account for the complex ways people enact information systems of all sorts into their social endeavors to accomplish organizational tasks. Sociomateriality has been referred to as an umbrella approach (Jones 2013, p. 2) because it points to encompasses a diverse set of research by a range of prominent scholars, such as "mangle of practice" (Pickering 1993), "human-machine configurations" (Suchman 2007), "agential realism" (Barad 1996), "body multiple" (Mol 2002), and "actor-network-theory" (Latour 2005). While each of these research traditions has pertinent differences, they do have one thing in common: They share a common epistemology that technology cannot be understood outside of its social practice, since the materiality of technology is shaped by practices and becomes part of these while simultaneously shaping the practices themselves. Originally inspired by Garfinkel's ethnomethodology (Garfinkel 1991) ethnographic research within CSCW (Harper 2000; Randall et al. 2007; Crabtree et al. 2012) provides essential stepping-stones in terms of understanding collaborative work have led to major impacts in the design of technology research. Building on this tradition, and the extended work, we, in this book, are in particular inspired by Suchman's perspective on sociomateriality, as it appears in the added chapters on reconfiguration and mutual constitutions in the second edition of her book, now entitled Human-Machine reconfigurations. She writes:

> This intimate co-constitution of configured materialities with configuring agencies clearly implies a very different understanding of the human-machine interface. Read in association with the empirical investigations of complex sociomaterial sites described above, 'the interface' becomes the name for a category of contingently enacted cuts occurring always within sociomaterial practices, that effect 'person' and 'machine' as distinct entities, and that in turn enable particular forms of subject-object intra-actions. At the same time, the singularity of 'the interface' explodes into a multiplicity of more or less closely aligned, dynamically configured moments of encounter within sociomaterial configurations, objectified as persons and machines. (Suchman 2007, p. 268)

Sociomateriality specifies that when we study the technical artefact, it cannot be understood outside of the practices in which it becomes enacted. The boundaries of what makes the technical artefact are shaped by the practices in which it is used. But, how do we take into account all of these sociomaterial phenomena—in all their complexity—when faced with the task of designing information technology? In other words, how can a sociomaterial perspective inform the design of digital artefacts?

Research involved in designing digital artefacts is also diverse and includes "activity theory" (Nardi 1996), "participatory design" (Simonsen and Robertsen 2013), "contextual design" (Beyer and Holtzblatt 1997), "distributed cognition" (Hutchins 1995), "complex mediation" (Bødker and Andersen 2005), "intrinsic practice transformation" (Kaptelinin and Bannon 2012), "imbrication" (Leonardi 2011), and "cooperative design" (Greenbaum and Kyng 1991; Schmidt 2011). While each stream of research is different, they all build upon the fundamental understanding that the material matters and social practices of the domain we design for are of the most importance when designing the material properties of artefacts. This insight has led to the emergence of ethnographic techniques in diverse types of technology design methods (e.g. Bødker et al. 2004; Randall et al. 2007; Blomberg and Karasti 2013), and the close-to-established standard of exploring the practices one is designing for before engaging with design activities.

In this book, the healthcare field serves as the focus area for design. Thus, our conceptualization of sociomaterial-design is built upon our efforts in exploring the practices and technologies in healthcare practices as an exemplary domain. Health-care as a domain for design has received attention in several information technology research fields such as health informatics (Reddy et al. 2011; Bjørn and Kensing 2013), CSCW (Bansler and Kensing 2010; Fitzpatrick and Ellingsen 2013), CHI (Tang and Carpendale 2007; Park and Chen 2012), and IS (Braa et al. 2004; David-son and Chiasson 2005). Despite their differences, common interests can be found across these diverse fields and many researchers publish across the disciplinary boundaries. Thus, when we refer in this book to the design domain of healthcare, we join scholars with an interest in designing for healthcare based upon in-depth under-standing of the practices (e.g. Ellingsen and Monteiro 2003; Bardram and Bossen 2005; Andersen et al. 2010; Tentori et al. 2012). The common interest is to design, build, and provide technological artefacts that support the work of people and their practices in healthcare. However if technological artefacts *are made* in multiple complex sociomaterial practices, and therefore do not have pre-determined bound-aries, how can we then design such artefacts? How can you design a "sociomaterial artefact" without pre-determined boundaries?

The fundamental difference between sociomateriality and design is that socio-materiality is an ontological approach, while design is a practical concern for how to build useful technical artefacts. Some might claim that the two are epistemologi-cally so far from each other that it is not possible unite them. Due to the interest in introducing the complexities of technical artefacts (e.g. Bijker et al. 1987) through analytical explorations of the past and history of artefacts, sociomateriality research has a tendency to be perceived as looking back rather than forward by design re-searchers. On the other hand, when design research explores an interest in interven-tion and change through technological innovations (e.g. Johannesen et al. 2013), sociomaterial researchers have a tendency to refer to the process as having a tech-nologically deterministic perspective. We, the authors of this book, are ourselves part of both communities and strongly believe that the sociomaterial interest does not need to entail interest in historical explorations, nor that design interventions are always technologically deterministic. Instead, we strongly believe that it is possible to create an interventionist design agenda based upon the sociomaterial ontology of complexity. The goal with this book is, thus, to explain what *sociomaterial-design* is in such a way that researchers from the diverse communities of sociomateriality and design can come together to take the next steps in producing technologies that will take into account the cross-sections of sociomaterial practices. We do this by building upon the work of Suchman (Suchman 2007), while introducing the con-cept of *bounding*. Briefly, bounding refer to the temporal practice by which artefacts are enacted in sociomaterial practices, through binding together artefacts, locations, and movements in diverse ways while setting the boundaries for what is inside or outside the sociomaterial entity at different points in time.

In this book, we bring together several bodies of literature that take *practice* (Schatzki 2012) as their point of departure. First, *sociomateriality* offers a relational ontology that allows us to account for the constitutively entangled nature of arte-facts, people, and practices. The notion of sociomateriality refers to the entwined nature of the social and the material. The two are inseparably, constitutively entan-gled. Sociomateriality highlights the nexus of doings, materialities, and discourses that people carefully enact. It offers an analytical perspective from which neither artefacts, nor people, nor practices are seen naked and alone, revealing solely their inherent properties. Instead, people, artefacts, and practices are bound together into one entity within networks or assemblages with dynamic boundaries. Second, *de-sign research* strives to draw theoretical approaches into the practices of designing digital artefacts to ensure that work practices and digital artefacts remain syner-gistic—even after the initial disruption of work practices when new technological artefacts are introduced. Understanding practice with the aim of designing, imple-menting, and adapting digital artefacts to be enacted in particular organizational practices is a critical path crucial for design research, and we believe that the so-ciomaterial agenda can help this path along. However, we have still not solved the problem of how to approach design of technological artefacts while preserving the ontological understanding of sociomateriality.

We find the sociomaterial perspective to be an intriguing and challenging con-nection with design, since interesting questions arise, such as "How can we design technical artefacts without pre-determined boundaries?" Our aim is to theoretically and empirically investigate what it means to design technological artefacts while embracing the multiplicity of practices that occur when practitioners engage with technologies in practice. Bringing sociomateriality and design together creates a new entity, a new way to think about both sociomateriality and design, namely sociomaterial-design. Sociomaterial-design concerns an approach to design where we, as sociomaterial-designers, *investigate current* information systems and *design future* artefacts while insisting on an open-ended understanding of where the bound-aries for our "object" begin and end. What makes the artefact we study and the artefact we design is not pre-assumed, but instead understood as an emergent phe-nomenon. We use the hyphenated nomenclature sociomaterial-design to emphasize our interdisciplinary interest and explicitly distance ourselves from sharp disciplin-ary boundaries between the two. By binding the two distinctly different disciplinary interests together with the hyphen, we underline that we do not just seek to bring the sociomaterial ontology to design, nor do we simply bring the design agenda to the sociomaterial literature. Instead, we create a new form of entity, where both intra-act.

The title of the book is *Sociomaterial-Design: Bounding Technologies in Prac-tice*, and the word "bounding" plays a central role in the theoretical argument and practical application of sociomaterial-design. When we remove the pre-determined boundaries from the artefacts we study and design, we need a new vocabulary that makes it possible for us as sociomaterial-designers to refer to the practices by which boundaries are made, changed, moved, and taken away in the constantly fluctuat-ing engagement with artefacts. "Bounding" serves our purpose, since becoming bounded has a double meaning—namely to bind together, as in a hyphenated-structure, and to set the boundaries for what makes the entity, as in [bracketing structures]. "Bounding technologies in practices" thus refers to the practices by which artefacts are enacted in practice, binding together social-material practices and multiple artefacts in dynamic ways, while creating new dynamic entities by bracketing out what is in and what is out at certain times. Our book unfolds what "bounding technologies in practice" entails as part of the practices of sociomaterial-designers.

Working in interdisciplinary research institutions and projects for the last 10 years, we have seen how a divide can be created between researchers with a theoretical interest in *unpacking* the complexities of practices and researchers with a design agenda who seek to *reduce* the complexity of practice to be able to design artefacts. Our aim with this book is to enter conversations with both sets of audiences, using empirical cases in healthcare practices and illustrative examples for how to enact sociomaterial-design in practice. We have chosen to engage with the two audiences by identifying them as two fictional characters based upon our own experiences and engagement with researchers from the different disciplines. We have created the characters as generic figures that can ask each other questions and seek to learn from each other throughout the book. It is important to note that any direct resemblance with real people is coincidental. The two characters are Alan and Ada.

Ada and Alan

Alan is 45 years old, married, and has two children ages 9 and 11. He has been in research for 20 years, the last 5 years as professor in science and technology studies. Alan has a theoretical interest in the complexities in practice, and has in the last 10 years studied nurses' work in hospitals. His approach is to conduct ethnographic open-ended empirical investigations of medical practice, in which he spends many hours observing the practice. He focuses on particularly surprising phenomena that may occur and explores these in detail. Alan mostly publishes his work in books or in social science journals; however, at times he also participates in medical conferences to inspire his work. He has published and contributed to research about concerns for patient safety, technology politics in hospitals, and gender figurations in hospital work. *What drives Alan's research are the surprising complexities revealed when engaging with healthcare practices.*

Ada is 45 years old, married, and has two children ages 12 and 14. She is a professor in computer science, with a specialty in software development. During the last 10 years, she has focused on healthcare systems, since she wanted to make a difference in a domain she cares about. She mostly publishes in ACM (Association for Computing Machinery) conference proceedings, but also attends medical conferences to inspire her work. Ada works with users when designing information systems to support their work, entailing close collaboration with medical doctors. Her approach is to find a problem faced by the users and to design a solution. Ada has excellent technical skills and, together with her team, she designs, develops, and implements technical solutions for the healthcare practice. In certain instances, Ada also engages the healthcare industry in her projects, in order to move from prototypes to products that will be continuously used. Examples of systems that

Fig. 1.1 Mock-up whiteboard to determine the
location of a new digital
whiteboard in an Emergency
Department

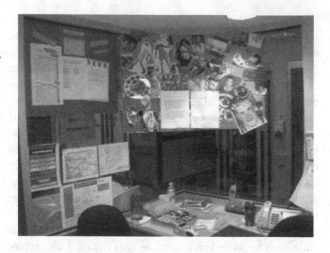

Ada creates include digital whiteboards and modules for chronic illness in electronic medical records. *What drives Ada's research are the shifting set of problems
experienced by the user in practice and how to figure out how new design material
(e.g., sensors, fabric, sound, and light) can be utilized in the design of ubiquitous
computing that supports technical solutions to concrete problems.*

Ada and Alan both want to keep extending their perspectives on their research,
as well as challenge each other's work to test if expanding their horizons could
lead them to new, unexpected ways to solve the same basic problem. Their shared
core interest is to have excellent medical practices and technologies in hospitals.
However, when they occasionally meet at medical conferences, they have problems
relating to each other's work directly. Despite finding each other's work fascinating
and appealing, they have trouble applying any surprising new insights in their own
research. This book is written with Ada and Alan as the shared audience in mind,
which means that some part of the book might be completely new for Alan, but will
seem as basic knowledge for Ada and vice versa. Working interdisciplinarily is not
unique in the area of human agency and technologies, and as such we humbly join
others with the same interest in exploring the intersections between academic fields.

Bringing together the interests of Ada and Alan, we, provide in this book rich, con-
text-dense empirical examples from our two longitudinal studies of healthcare work
in EDs. In this way, the book exercises what has been called the next frontier of sociomaterial research, namely to unpack sociomaterial practices *across contexts* (Gaskin
et al. 2013). To our knowledge very few researchers (Balka et al. 2008; Boulus and
Bjørn 2008) have taken up the challenge of conducting analytical comparisons across
qualitative longitudinal empirical cases in healthcare, so the book is unique in that respect. Our two cases are particularly relevant for demonstrating the sociomaterial-design approach, since both cases comprise rich data material about how the healthcare
practices went through processes of digitalization over the periods of the two studies.
In this way, the empirical cases have direct interest for both Alan and Ada (Fig. 1.1).

The two cases both took place in North American (the United States and Canada)
within two pediatric EDs. Throughout this book, we will draw from these empirical
cases when demonstrating the intersections between sociomateriality and design,

and how these fields *together* can reach much more nuanced understandings of organizational practice in general and healthcare practice in particular. These understandings can serve as the foundation for design of digital systems.

The book is structured into three main sections. The first section, "Theoretical Perspective," introduces the history and concepts of practices, sociomateriality, and design. The second section, "Empirical Perspective," brings forward the method, empirical cases, examples, and comparative analysis that unite our two empirical cases. The third section, "Sociomaterial-Design," brings together literature and empirical findings to articulate the concept of bounding practices. It is in this final part of the book that we elaborate on our approach of how to create design interventions based upon the sociomaterial epistemology.

References

Andersen T., Bjørn P., et al.: Designing for collaborative interpretation in telemonitoring: reintroducing patients as diagnostic agents. Int. J. Med. Inform. (2010). doi:10.1016/j.ijmedinf.2010.09.010

Balka, E., Bjørn P., et al.: Steps towards a typology for health informatics. In: Computer Supported Cooperative Work (CSCW), San Diego, CA, USA, ACM 2008

Bansler, J., Kensing F.: Information infrastructure for health care: Connecting practices across institutional and professional boundaries. CSCW Int. J. **19**, 519–520 (2010)

Barad, K.: Meeting the universe halfway: Realism and social constructivism without contradiction. In: Nelson L. H., Nelson J. (eds.) Feminism, Science, and the Philosophy of Science, pp. 161–194. Kluwer, London (1996)

Bardram, J., Bossen C.: Mobility work: the spatial dimension of collaboration at a hospital. CSCW Int. J. **14**, 131–160 (2005)

Berg, M.: Rationalizing Medical Work: Decision-Support Techniques and Medical Practices. MIT Press, Cambridge (1997)

Beyer, H., Holtzblatt K.: Contextual Design: Defining Customer-Centered Systems, Elsevier, Amsterdam (1997)

Bijker, W., Hughes, T., et al.: The Social Construction of Technological Systems: New Directions in the Sociology and Historiy of Technology. MIT Press, Cambridge (1987)

Bjørn, P., Kensing F.: Special issue on information infrastructures for healthcare: the global and local relation. Int. J. Med. Inform. **82**, 281–282 (2013)

Blomberg, J., Karasti H.: Reflections on 25 years or ethnography in CSCW. CSCW Int. J. **22**, 373–423 (2013)

Bødker, S.: Through the Interface: A Human Activity Approach to User Interface Design. Lawrence Erlbaum, Mahwah (1991)

Bødker, S., Andersen P.B.: Complex mediation. Hum. Computer Interact. **20**, 353–402 (2005)

Bødker, K., Kensing F., et al.: Participatory IT Design: Designing for Business and Workplace Realities. MIT Press, Cambridge (2004)

Boulus, N., Bjørn P.: A cross-case analysis of technology-in-use practices: EPR-adaptation in Canada and Norway. Int. J. Med. Inform. **79**(6), 97–108 (2008)

Bowker, G.C., Star S.L.: Sorting Things Out: Classification and its Consequences. MIT Press, Cambridge (2002)

Braa, J., Monterio E., et al.: Networks of action: sustainable health information systems across developing countries. MIS Q. **28**(3), 337–362 (2004)

Crabtree, A., Rouncefield M., et al.: Doing Design Ethnography. Springer, Berlin (2012)

Davidson, E., Chiasson M.: Contextual influences on technology use mediation: a comparative analysis of electronic medical record systems. Eur. J. Inf. Syst. **14**, 6–18 (2005)

Dourish, P.: Where the Action is: The Foundations of Embodied Interaction. MIT Press, Cambridge (2004)

Ellingsen, G., Monteiro E.: A patchwork planet integration and cooperation in hospitals. CSCW Int. J. **12**(1), 71–95 (2003)

Fitzpatrick, G., Ellingsen G.: A review of 25 years of CSCW research in healthcare: contributions, challenges and future agendas. CSCW Int. J. **22**, 609–665 (2013)

Garfinkel, H.: Studies in Ethnomethodology. Wiley, Hoboken (1991). (orginally published by Prentice Hall in 1967)

Gaskin, J., Berente, N., et al.: Towards generalizable sociomaterial inquiry: a computational approach for zooming in and out of sociomaterial routines. MIS Q. **38**(3), 849–871 (2013)

Greenbaum, J., Kyng M.: Design at Work: Cooperative Design of Computer Systems. Routledge, London (1991)

Harper, R.: The organisation in ethnography. CSCW Int. J. **9**, 239–264 (2000)

Hutchins, E.: Cognition in the Wild. MIT Press, Cambridge (1995)

Johannesen, L.K., Obstfelder A., et al.: Scaling of an information system in a public healthcare market–Infrastructuring from the vendor's perspective. Int. J. Med. Inform. **82**, 180–188 (2013)

Jones, M.: A matter of life and death: Exploring conceptualizations of sociomateriality in the context of critcal care. MIS Q. **38**(3), 895–925 (2013)

Kaptelinin, V., Bannon L.: Interaction design beyond the product: creating technology-enhanded activity spaces. Hum. Computer Interact. **27**(3), 277–309 (2012)

Latour, B.: Reassemling the Social: An Introduction to Actor-Network-Theory. Oxford University Press, Oxford (2005)

Law, J.: After Method: Mess is Social Science Research. Routledge, London (2004)

Leonardi, P.: When flexible routines meet flexible technologies: affordance, constraint, and the imbrication of human and material agencies. MIS Q. **35**(1), 147–167 (2011)

Leonardi, P., Nardi, B., et al.: Materiality and Organizing: Social Interaction in a Technological World. Oxford Press, Oxford (2012)

Mol, A.: The Body Multiple: Ontology in Medical Practice. Duke University Press, London (2002)

Nardi, B.: Context and Consciousness: Activity Theory and Human Computer Interaction. MIT Press, Cambridge (1996)

Orlikowski, W.: Sociomaterial practices: exploring technology at work. Organ. Stud. **28**(9), 1435–1448 (2007)

Park, S.Y., Chen Y.: Adaptation as design: learning from an EMR deployment study. Computer Human Interaction, Austin, Texas, USA, ACM, pp. 2097–2106 (2012)

Pickering, A.: The mangle of practice: agency and emergence in the sociology of science. Am. J. Sociol. **99**(3), 559–589 (1993)

Randall, D., Harper, R., et al.: Fieldwork for Design: Theory and Practice. Springer, London (2007)

Reddy, M., Gorman, P., et al.: Special issue on supporting collaboration in healthcare settings: the role of informatics. Int. J. Med. Inform. **80**(8), 541–543 (2011)

Schatzki, T.: A primer on practice. In: Higgs J., et al. (eds.) Practice-Based Education: Perspectives and Strategies. Sense Publishers, Rotterdam (2012)

Schmidt, K.: Cooperative Work and Coordinative Practices: Contributions to the Conceptual Foundations of Computer-Supported Cooperative Work (CSCW). Springer, London (2011)

Simonsen, J., Robertsen T.: Routledge International Handbook of Participatory Design. Routledge: Taylor & Francis Group, London (2013)

Suchman, L.: Human-Machine Reconfigurations: Plans and Situated Actions. Cambridge University Press, Cambridge (2007)

Tang, C., Carpendale S.: An observational study on information flow during nurses' shift change. CHI. San Jose, CA, USA, ACM, pp. 219–228 (2007)

Tentori, M., Hayes G., et al.: Pervasive computering for hospital, chronic, and preventive care. Found. Trends Hum. Computer Interact. **5**(1), 1–95 (2012)

Part I
Theoretical Perspective

Chapter 2
Sociomateriality & Design

The aim of this book is to create a theoretical foundation for how we can combine the insights from sociomateriality with the interests of design and vice versa. This mean that we need to start to unpack both sociomateriality and design to study their foundations and then identify a common ground to create the new entity of Sociomaterial-Design. In this chapter we will introduce sociomateriality and design, while identifying the common ground between these—namely the practice-based interest.

2.1 Practice

A deep-seated concern for *practice* unites sociomaterial scholarship and design research despite their stark differences in analytical level, scope, and audience. Following "the practice turn" (Schatzki et al. 2001; Reckwitz 2002) the concept of practice refers to a nexus of doings, artefacts, and sayings carried by a specific form of practical understanding. Going beyond people's mere doings, a practice lens highlights the routinized and performative character of actions in which objects are constituted, bodies shaped, subjects treated, and the world is understood. But what is practice and what is the practice approach? Reckwitz (2002) makes a distinction between "practice" (praxis), meaning the "whole of human action," and "a practice" (praktik), which is a particular type of "routinized behavior," and our concern here is the latter (Reckwitz 2002, pp. 249–250). The practice approach is thus about exploring people's routinized behavior when engaged in practice. The practice approach specifies that we cannot open up people's heads and look inside to see what they think and, as such, there are distinct differences between cognitive science and the practice approach. However, the reluctance to open up people's heads does *not* mean that practice research refuses to think about mental activities. Quite to the contrary, mental activities are very important in practice research. The practice approach insists that mental and bodily activities cannot be meaningfully separated, but instead comprise one entity in which people perform the routinized bodily/mentally activities, making the practice. This means that we do not have access to "see"

© Springer International Publishing Switzerland 2014   15
P. Bjørn, C. Østerlund, *Sociomaterial-Design,* Computer Supported Cooperative Work,
DOI 10.1007/978-3-319-12607-4_2

what people think, but instead have to study how their mental activities become manifested in practice. The bodily activities are, thus, mental activities at the same time and when we study practice, we study both together. A practice is a "routinized way in which bodies are moved, objects are handled, subjects are treated, things are described, and the world is understood" (Reckwitz 2002, p. 250). Practice is immediately social, meaning that behavior and understanding—which appear in practice—are carried out by multiple different bodies/minds that together form the routinized engagement. People might be placed at different locations or at different points in time, but still share a practice together. When practice conceptually consists of both bodily and mental activities, there cannot be any rigorous distinction between what is "inside" or "outside" the mind and body (Ibid, p. 252). When we learn how to engage in social practices, we enter particular communities of practices (Wenger 1998) that have particular routinized behaviors for the inclusive bodies/minds that are already members. Entering a practice is thus a process where learners move from legitimate peripheral participation towards full participation (Lave and Wenger 1991), which is a product of the training the body/mind in certain ways.

> Practices are routinized bodily activities: as interconnected complexes of behavioral acts they are movements of the body. A social practice is the product of training the body in certain way: when we learn a practice we learn to be bodies in a certain way. (Reckwitz 2002, p. 251)

Practice is what practitioners do. Practice is the professional engagement, performed repeatedly and regularly by practitioners to establish or maintain proficiency within professional fields. Learning the "rules of practice in any given community entails a series of encounters with objects involved in the practice" including tools, texts, technologies, and symbols (Bowker and Star 2002, p. 294). Members of communities of practice develop together a shared repertoire of resources, or a shared practice, that are used when participants engage in practice and perform their activities. Creating the shared repertoire takes time and requires engagement from the practitioners in terms of participation and negotiation (Wenger 1998). Referring to Heidegger, the Dreyfus brothers (Dreyfus 1997) discuss skillful practitioners' engagements with artefacts in practice. They write: "In our normal everyday coping we deal with ready-to-hand equipment without any thought at all. This skillful dealing may be general and routine, but, as our skill model makes clear, it can be as specific and subtle as the response of a chess grandmaster to a complex chess position" (Dreyfus 1997, p. 27).

When we investigate a practice (e.g., healthcare practice) with the aim of designing for that practice, we do it to "dismantle the common-sense conceptions of cooperative work, take them apart, unpack and disclose the hidden practices of articulation work, and thus give us access—analytically and conceptually—to the intricate ways and means of the production of social order in cooperative activities" (Schmidt 2011, p. 4). Investigating practice includes unpacking what might go unnoticed by the practitioners, however hugely important those practices could be for the fundamental structure of the work (Star and Strauss 1999), while carefully being aware of the possible impact (both positive and negative) of us shedding light on these formerly opaque practices (Suchman 1995).

Artefacts and objects take important parts in practice. Routinized practices do in many situations include professional embodied engagement with multiple artefacts. Entering the ED, we quickly notice the wide range of artefacts (analog as well as digital) that are part of the routinized practices that are the work of the healthcare professionals. Artefacts are "necessary components of many practices—just as indispensable as bodily and mental activities" (Reckwitz 2002, p. 252). Technologies are embedded parts of practice. Studying practice must take into consideration the "routinized body/knowledge/things-patterns" which together makes the entity (Reckwitz 2002).

> Routinized social practices occur in the sequence of time, in repetition; social order is thus basically social production. For practice theory, then, the 'breaking' and 'shifting' of structures must take place in everyday crises of routines, in constellations of interpretative interdeterminacy and of the inadequacy of knowledge with which the agent, carrying out a practice, is confronted in the face of a 'situation.' (Reckwitz 2002, p. 255)

When we refer in this book to "practice" as part of our analysis, we refer to two types of professional practice: *research practice* and *healthcare practice*. Since one of our purposes in writing this book is to illuminate the interdisciplinary research practice of sociomaterial-design, we have an explicit interest in *research practices*, as does the work that Ada and Alan do. When we talk about research practice, we are referring to the activities of Ada and Alan reading books, journals, and research papers; discussing their work with others; writing their research; and analyzing data and design technologies, in addition to the other activities that go into the varied practice of academic research. Research practice includes the practices by which Ada and Alan collect allies, both inside the laboratory and in society (Latour 1987). The aspect of Ada and Alan's research practice that concerns us in the book is the practice they interact with and research, namely healthcare practice. Because of their different disciplines and the particular natures of their research interests, Ada and Alan interact with the healthcare practice in different ways—and this divergence in interaction is where our interest resides. Ada and Alan are both professional experts in research practice and, despite their interdisciplinary differences, they share common repertoire of resources, even though the tools, texts, and symbols have different uses. Healthcare practice is the professional practice of healthcare workers involved with performing the activities of diagnosing, treating, and preventing illnesses. The healthcare practices that concern us in this book entail, in particular, the practices ongoing in EDs and, even more specifically, in the EDs of North American pediatric hospitals. However, while our interest here is specific, the findings we can draw from the studies are of a much more general nature and are applicable to other settings (see in particular the chapter titled "Sociomaterial-Design beyond Healthcare").

Practice, thus, in this book is the common denominator between sociomateriality and design and serves as the foundation on which we can build our new entity, sociomaterial-design. Sociomaterial research and the design research would not exist without the organizational practices that they strive to conceptualize and support. Without practice there would be little to design for and study, whether in the ED, the science lab, or on the stock exchange floor. In doing so, our analytical focus becomes the "shifting" and "breaking" of structures within the healthcare work when new technologies enter the scene and become part of what constitute the practice in emergency work. Alan and Ada are both directed at the practices produced by the medical infrastructure and setup of the hospital and they both share an interest in improving these practices, despite their very different approaches.

The *sociomaterial* literature builds on a relational ontology assuming that this *practice* nexus does not simply mediate *a priori* objects and subject, organizational structures, or rules. The entities found at the nexus of practice are not given in advance and carry no inherent properties (Orlikowski and Scott 2008). Rather, they are performed (Barad 2003) or enacted (Suchman 2007). The subject and object do not merely *inter*act by exerting force upon one another; instead they emerge out of their encounter through *intra*-actions. Following this line of thinking, practices are always both social *and* material—even purely discursive practices. In sociomaterial practices, the material phenomena are inseparable from the apparatus of bodily production (Haraway 1991; Suchman 2007, p. 286).

Design research strives explicitly to improve *practice* through the theory-driven design of information technology (IT) artefacts (Bannon and Bødker 1997; Aarts et al. 2007). While most designers do not subscribe to a praxiological approach as articulated in "the practice turn," they nevertheless approach practice as a nexus of doings, artefacts, and discourses enacted in routinized ways over time. This entails a process approach where the nexus is constantly being constructed and reconstructed as it is designed, built, sold, and used (Simonsen and Robertsen 2013). In this way "practice" is important for both Ada and Alan, and therefore can serve as the first element in the scaffolding that supports sociomaterial-design. Before we delve deeper into the literatures on sociomateriality and design, we need a second element to build our scaffold, namely the socio-technical research, which to this date has been critical in the development of the intersections between human agency and design (Fig. 2.1).

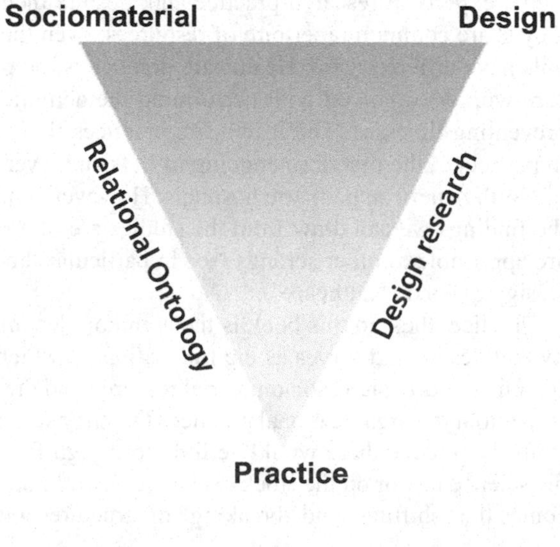

Fig. 2.1 Sociomaterial, Design, Practice

2.2   Socio-technical

When we are creating the links between the ontological understanding of sociomateriality and design, we need to think about a common ground on which the two distinct different disciplines can engage. Therefore, we need to re-visit the foundations on which technology design began to incorporate the social aspects of work within the agendas of design. We need to build upon our sociomaterial ontological understanding from this perspective. We need to address the design interest of fields such as computer-supported cooperative work (CSCW) and participatory design (PD) in the perspectives of sociomateriality. Basically, we will address the discussion that emerges when Alan meets Ada, and Alan begins explaining the sociomaterial agendas at the healthcare conferences that they both participate in.

When Alan starts to talk about the ontological foundation of sociomateriality with Ada, some of the concepts sound familiar, while others are totally new to her. The idea that technology and the social organization of work have to be understood as one is very familiar to Ada and a major part of the theoretical foundations of her work. Ada is used to labelling this approach the socio-technical approach to system design. However, in the discussions it is clear that Alan insists there is a difference between socio-technical approaches and sociomateriality. Therefore, let's start by investigating what the socio-technical approach entails.

> The story of socio-technical design is closely allied with action research. This is more a philosophy than a methodology. It describes a process and a humanistic set of principles that in our context is associated with technology and changes. It can be used to contribute to most problem-solving in work situations, providing that both the innovators and recipients are willing to use a democratic approach. (Mumford 2006, p. 317)

The socio-technical approach is more than 50 years old and was first introduced by The Tavistock Institute of Human Relations (Trist 1981), which also created the fundamental agenda behind action research (Rapoport 1970). Both the socio-technical approach and action research have been critical to the development of design research; for instance, these created the foundation for Soft Systems Methodology (Checkland and Holwell 1998) and Reflective System Development (Mathiassen 1998). What was special with The Tavistock Institute was that they engaged in the development of research with a strong link to practical circumstances in the world. Their interest began with immediate problem situations that they wanted to address while identifying and developing ways in which such situations can be solved at a more general level. One famous example is the desire of therapists and researchers to develop new methods to assist war-damaged soldiers in regaining their mental health and returning to civilian life (Mumford 2006, p. 319). In this case, researchers collaborated with therapists in developing new methods, while at the same time applying the methods in practice. This continuing interest in solving an immediate problem while also developing research is the basic premise for the socio-technical approach. Studies of workers and employees were strong during socio-technical research that occurred in the 1970s. One example is the study of the organization of work in mines and how changing the work situation impacted the miners' job satisfaction. Within the realm of wanting to impact the world in a positive way, the socio-technical approach was concerned with how employees, management, processes, and organizations interacted and how the material matter of the work matters for the workers (Leonardi et al. 2012, p. 39).

2.2.1   Socio-technical Approach to System Design

For many researchers in Scandinavia who aimed at involving workers as co-de-signers, the ontological understanding encompassed socio-technical approaches to system design (Mumford 2001)—thereby supporting workers' practices, as well as, simultaneously, democracy in work (Grudin 1988). The trade union perspective in the late 1970s and the 1980s was very influential in setting the groundwork for socio-technical system design (Mathiassen 1998). Many projects were completed that put bringing in the user and their practices as the main focal point (Carlsson et al. 1978; Bødker et al. 2000; Kensing et al. 2009). Besides focusing on the prac-tices of workers, the main research contribution that emerged from these projects included methods and processes for software development (Andersen et al. 1986; Bødker et al. 2004). Socio-technical approaches stressed job satisfaction, workers' needs, and skill enhancement—and the focus was to "embrace a user-oriented per-spective, by emphasizing that through insights into the work practices in which the IT application should be used and use that as the starting point for implementation" (Berg 1999, p. 89). The dominant driving forces were the aims to focus on demo-cratic approaches, including the user perspective, and to ensure that new technology enabled people, rather than constrained.

Along this approach, the focus on collaborative practice was very strong. Jona-than Grudin quoting Pelle Ehn, who was one of founding fathers of the Scandinavian approach to system design, said at the first CSCW conference in 1988: "All work is cooperative." The focus on the cooperative aspects of work, the political interest of workers, and the design of technology was critical in all sociotechnical approaches. Now the political interest in bringing in and pointing to the social organization of work and how it was important for system design also became in focus. This strong political agenda in system design came from the reaction to the artificial intelligence (AI) research and the office automation movement (e.g. Hammer 1990), where the focus was on the office procedure efficiency rather than on the satisfaction of the workers. So while CSCW grew out of AI and office automation (Krasner and Grief 1986), it also changed the focus from simple efficiency to include consideration of how people work and collaborate.

> CSCW should be conceived of as an endeavor to understand the nature and requirements of cooperative work with the objective of designing computer-based technologies for coopera-tive work arrangements. The fact that multiple individuals, situated in different work set-tings and situations, with different responsibilities, perspectives, and propensities, interact and are mutually dependent in the conduct of their work has important implications for the design of computer systems intended to support them in this effort. (Schmidt and Bannon 1992, p. 11)

Within the arena of CSCW, the combined design and sociomaterial agenda was introduced. Being an interdisciplinary research space, CSCW brought together design researchers and ethnographers with the aim of bringing the user perspective (still based upon the democratic agenda from socio-technical approaches) into the design. The most famous CSCW debate from its early years was about The Coor-dinator (Winograd and Flores 1986; Suchman 1994). At the first CSCW conference in 1986, Terry Winograd presented the design of The Coordinator, a new commu-nications system. Almost 30 years later, The Coordinator does not seem as novel a technology, but at that time it was one of the first collaborative technologies built on a theoretical notion of human cognition. The Coordinator is basically an email application that allows users to tag their messages with categories such as "request," "promise," or "offer," and by this practice make it easier for people to respond since their reason for interaction is made explicit (for more details see Flores et al. 1988). At the time, the design approach behind The Coordinator was unique in that it was designed based upon a theoretical understanding of how people communicate. In their book, *Understanding Computers and Cognition* (Winograd and Flores 1986), Terry Winograd and Fernando Flores expressed their approach to system design for communication technologies to be based upon the theories of Speech Act created by Austin (Ibid). While Winograd presented The Coordinator at the first CSCW conference, Lucy Suchman made a critical analysis of the basic foundation for system design that emerged through The Coordinator system. Suchman's argued that categories and artefacts have politics that become embedded within the design of cooperative systems, if based upon the categories of Speech Act (Suchman 1994). The debate on The Coordinator ended in a special issue of the journal of CSCW, in which well-known researchers were invited to comment (e.g. Grudin and Grinter 1995; Lynch 1995; Orlikowski 1995). However, the debate at that time focused more on the different approaches between ethnography and design, since it was then a huge interest for the community (Blomberg et al. 1993; Blomberg and Karasti 2013). The centre of the debate, thus, concerned the difficulties of embracing ethnography and design and bringing those together (Randall et al. 2007), rather than the fundamental discussion about the political impact of specific theoretical understanding in system design.

2.2.2 What Was Lost in the Coordinator Debate?

However, if we are to investigate the debate about The Coordinator more closely, we find a much more nuanced perspective and debate that is not related to ethnography and design as such, but instead to the ontological understanding of how we can understand technologies, organizations, and practices. This ontological perspective came from researchers involved in science and technology studies, fields that do not have a design interest *per se* but are concerned with the practices by which technologies are made and interact in the world (Akrich and Latour 1992; Bowker and Star 2002; Suchman 2007). This ontological understanding was the groundwork for what we refer to in this book as sociomateriality.

When Suchman argued that categories have politics, she was referring to Winner's (Winner 1986) inscripted artefacts, Latour's study of science (Latour 1987), and Haraway's cyborg (Haraway 1990). The critical questions in these types of studies include how technologies are made, and how we can trace technology back through history to show how it is not a casual process, but instead an actor network, that makes technology, people, and organizations. Few have revisited this argument about politics in collaborative systems within the CSCW design community (Bjørn and Balka 2007a) and, in general, the argument about politics and technologies tends to be neglected when we talk about system design. Therefore, if we are

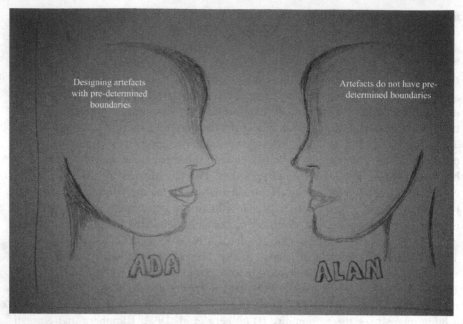

Fig. 2.2 Pre-determined boundaries

to bring together sociomateriality and design, we need to re-introduce the design audience to the debate about politics, entanglements, people, organizations, and technology (Fig. 2.2).

2.3 Sociomateriality

Sociomateriality refers to a particular epistemological and ontological understanding of technologies, people, and organizations. It stipulates that people and technologies are constitutively entangled and, to investigate technology, we need to attend to these entanglements in order to then explore the temporal meaning, boundaries, and properties that such technologies entail (Cecez-Kecmanovic et al. 2011). Sociomateriality emphasizes the *importance of material properties* of artefacts and the changes in social practices caused by enacting such technologies. Sociomateriality points to the *inseparability* of the social and the material. What is material and what is social cannot easily be determined, instead they are each part of the same phenomenon, meaning that what is social is also material and vice versa. If we are to study one or the other, we have to also explore how they are related. This leads to the next important characteristic of sociomateriality, namely *relational ontology*. Since we cannot separate the social and the material, we are required to study how they perform together in practice; essentially, how they are intertwined and entangled in practice. Sociomateriality, thus, specifies that the study of technology is also concerned with the study of *performativity* of artefacts in practice. By exploring performativity, the relational aspects of the sociomaterial entity emerge from its inseparability and the importance of the material properties becomes salient.

While we here provide an introduction to sociomateriality as one coherent approach, it is important to mention that many dispute what makes "materiality" and, thus, debates on sociomateriality are currently ongoing. Does materiality constitute the artefacts, the tangible, the machine, and the nonhuman; or is it the social, the human, the people, and the organization; or, rather, is it the work? And depending upon what it is made of, how can we—and how should we—then study its relations to performativity? Should we study the relations as "the mangle of practice" (Pickering 1995), as "imbrication" (Leonardi 2011), or as "intrinsic practices" (Kaptelinin and Bannon 2012)? Adding to the complexity are the distinct differences between how we can understand materiality of the physical artefact compared with how we can understand digital technologies. Some researchers argue that not all technologies have physical presence (Kallinikos et al. 2013), while others insist that the opposite is true. This inconsistency in the definition of the material properties of technological artefacts makes it difficult to point to sociomateriality as a stable approach; however, it is hoped that this book will play a part in stabilizing sociomateriality. It is not the purpose of this book to unfold all the diverse perspectives on sociomateriality (for an discussion of the diverse perspective we would suggest reading Leonardi and Barley 2010; Jones 2013). Instead the purpose of this book is to explain and demonstrate the fundamentals of sociomaterial-design. Therefore, we will reduce the discussions on sociomateriality to what is required only to establish what the term entails in relation to sociomaterial-design.

The sociomateriality part of sociomaterial-design builds fundamentally upon the work of Lucy Suchman, who is often quoted for her coining of the term sociomateriality (Jones 2013). Since we leave the sociotechnical agenda in Suchman's hands through her influential work in CSCW (Suchman 1983), we start our examination of sociomateriality by exploring the chapters added in the 2007 reprint (Suchman 2007) of her book, *Plans and Situated Actions* (Suchman 1987). Suchman's work is interdisciplinary and, argumentatively, has had a huge impact on design the fields such as CSCW, PD, and CHI—making her book a perfect point of departure for sociomateriality and design. While Suchman herself views her work as social science (Suchman 2007, introduction), she provides the capacity to make her work relevant for design, and this provision has been highly appreciated in much design literature (Dourish 2004, p. 70 ff.).

2.3.1 Figurations

Suchman's sociomaterial perspective on design takes its starting point in the figuration of the "user." When we study the practice of designing technology then, at its core, we find the concept of the "user" (Wilkie and Michael 2009), and if we then dive into the conceptualization of the "user," it becomes clear that the "user" is a figuration (Haraway 1990) created by the designers with the aim of getting insights in the "practices of future use" (Suchman 2007). However, if we are to crack open the figuration of the "user," it becomes evident that the people in practices are so much more than a "user" (Bannon et al. 2012). People are much more than their relation to a technology. "'The user' singularizes what is actually a multiplicity and fails to differentiate actors with very different relations to a given artefact" (Suchman 2007, p. 188). If we are to really comprehend the complexities of what we are designing for, we have to reformulate the question: Instead of only defining the "user" through personas or other participatory design techniques, we must concentrate on "the incorporation of the user into the sociomaterial assemblage that comprises a functioning machine" (Suchman 2007, p. 190). Likewise, technologies are also figural, as in made up of tropes and turns of phrase (Suchman 2007, refering to Haraway), which remind us of particular associations of meaning and practice. Technologies are thus forms of materialized figurations, in that they bring together assemblages of meaning and practice in a temporal mode between stabilization and unstable arrangements (Suchman 2007, p. 227). Figurations are dynamic and change form depending upon the multiple practices they engage with. Several empirical studies within healthcare demonstrate this point, for example the study of multiplicity in the diagnosis and treatment of atherosclerosis (Mol 2002) and the study of "cyborg hearts" in telemonitoring of patients with implantable cardioverter defibrillators (Bjørn and Markussen 2013).

This does not mean that we cannot stabilize technologies—we sure can. However, the technology will only be stable in particular figuration at particular time and then will change again at a later time. This ever-changing dynamic is critical for technologies to act as standards bringing together heterogeneous practices, since "every form of stabilization includes (…) the presence of instability" (Suchman 2007, p. 196). Thus, sociomateriality as part of sociomaterial-design forms a theoretical agenda that refuses to separate what is social from what is material; instead, sociomateriality stipulates that all practices are co-constituted by the social *and* the material. Therefore, we need to address our understanding of practice in terms of assemblages and entanglements—which we cannot separate, but instead have to study as they emerge in temporal practice.

2.3.2   Relational Ontology

This insistence on the relational ontology is not the same as saying that people and technologies only exist in relation to each other (Orlikowski and Scott 2008; Jones 2013). The lone computer shut down and disconnected from all sorts of digital networks and infrastructures still does exist. The point is that to encapsulate the sociomateriality of the computer, we must study the sociomaterial practices, which only emerge in practice where the agency of both the human and the technology operate together. The answer to the question, as to *when* this relational agency emerges between the human and the material artefact, is that this relation emerges in sociomaterial practice. It is in the practice that technologies and humans emerge and become relational and intertwined. However, when we as designers seek to design new technological artefacts, the distinction between the computer as the disconnected entity and the sociomaterial practices of the computer becomes only an analytical separation, which we do not have access to study. We never design, create, and build technologies as disconnected entities, and, as such, we should continuously remind ourselves of the relational characteristics of artefacts.

Sociomateriality builds upon the work of Suchman (2007) and Mol (2002), but has really been promoted by Wanda Orlikowski in information systems and organizational studies (Orlikowski and Scott 2008; Orlikowski 2010). Sociomateriality is thus an emergent research theme for many researchers interested in organization and technologies, and has received much attention in the last couple of years in the form of for instance, special issues (Cecez-Kecmanovic et al. 2011) and edited volumes (Leonardi et al. 2012). Understanding technologies in the perspective of social entanglements is not new *per se*. Within the research fields of the social studies of science, these discussions have been going on for years (Barad 1996; Law 2004; Latour 2005). However, what is new is how the sociomaterial research agenda becomes re-introduced and re-created within the interdisciplinary interest of information systems and design (Bjørn 2012; Bratteteig and Verne 2012; Kautz and Jensen 2012; Gaskin et al. 2013; Mazmanian et al. 2014). Mazmanian et al. (2014) re-introduce and demonstrate how Haraway's figuration (1991) and Suchman's reconfiguration (2007) can be used to illuminate the sociomaterial practices within planetary exploration, and suggest that the vocabulary of dynamic reconfigurations emphasizes the constant dynamic and inter-changeable intra-action between the social and the material (Mazmanian et al. 2014). Faraj and Azad (2012) dive into the literature on affordances and suggest expanding the concept of affordance to include the sociomaterial nexus in order to clarify and extend the boundary conditions of particular technologies (Faraj and Azad 2012). Bratteteig and Verne (2012) conduct a sociomaterial analysis of the work of phone service workers working in tax administration in Sweden, and demonstrate how the concept of imbrication helps illuminate the sociomaterial assemblages in their particular case (Bratteteig and Verne 2012). While each of these studies is interesting on its own terms, our interest here is to dig a little deeper into the ontological understanding of sociomateriality and how it can be related to design.

Putting sociomateriality on the agenda for information systems research has been driven by the collective interest of considering the material properties of the IT artefact in organizational studies (Orlikowski and Iacono 2001). The argument is that the focus on the IT artefact has been forgotten in organizational research in the last 10 years, and that this creates potentially problematic and unbalanced perspectives and findings within the related fields of study (Chiasson and Davidson 2009). Sociomateriality is thus a way to re-introduce the material matters of artefacts into the field of organizational research. While we agree overall with the agenda of including the material properties of IT artefacts in organizational research, our mission with this book is different. Instead of debating the material matters of artefacts in organizations, we are interested in showing how the sociomaterial agenda can engage with design.

To date, publications on sociomateriality have placed great emphasis on the ontological and epistemological framing of the topic (Mol 2002; Barad 2003; Suchman 2007; Orlikowski and Scott 2008). The goal has been to develop an ontological and epistemological position that allows us to explore the relations among the material (e.g., IT systems) and the social without privileging one over the other. Sociomateriality is an "opportunity to move beyond the privileging or either the social or the material" (Jones 2013, p. 3). Classic information systems theories tend to promote ontological and epistemological positions that fall into either a material determinism, overemphasizing the material, or an ideological voluntarism, favoring the social (Leonardi and Barley 2008). Sociomaterial approaches articulate a position that allows us to explore the entanglement of the material *and* the social. Across this body of work we find a preoccupation with the entwined and entangled nature of sociomaterial phenomena. The image of something knotty, entwined, and entangled refers to both common empirical observations and a shared relational ontology.

In the field, many sociomaterial scholars find that it makes little sense to examine one artefact at a time when, in fact, reality presents an entanglement of sociomaterial relations. Figuring out where one begins and another ends can be difficult, if not meaningless. Ontologically, some sociomaterial researchers reject the idea that people and artefacts exist in and of themselves with separately attributable properties. The social and the material are ontologically inseparable or, in Barad's (2003) words, they are "constitutive entanglements." We cannot presume they are independent or interdependent entities with distinct or inherent properties. What takes its place is a relational ontology insisting that relations come first. In Mol's words, "to be is to be related" (Mol 2002, p. 54). Artefacts and people alike acquire their forms, attributes, and capabilities through their intra-actions, not through inherent properties. People and things start out and forever remain in relationships. Properties of an artefact are, thus, not intrinsically features of that artefact; rather, those features obtain analytical significance only in relation to and by way of contrast with other artefacts and people over time. Consequently, the properties and boundaries of sociomaterial artefacts are not ontological prior to this point. They become determinate only in their relations.

2.3.3   Ball of Yarn

But what do we do with a world all tangled up? What allows us to separate out and join together things in this knotty and entangled mess? Haraway (Haraway 1987; Haraway 1994) suggests that we approach this entwined ball of yarn by carefully studying particular strings and following these over time to see which relations the string creates. By pulling one string in the ball of yarn and carefully following it through time and history, we get insights into which relations are important for the sociomaterial practices we study. Barad (Barad 1996; Barad 2003; Barad 2007) extends the image of the entangled practice by introducing the notion of "agential cuts" to describe the work it takes for people to separate out and cut into shape these sociomaterial entanglements that originate from following the strings in the yarn.

Agential cuts perform separations between strings to consider or strings to cut, for what becomes inside or what becomes outside. Through agential actions, we create distinctions and order by bounding together elements into artefacts. This is not merely an epistemological exercise where people construct social meanings. Agential cuts are ontological. People build their world—artefacts, actions, and meanings. Barad (1996) argues "knowledge projects entail the drawing of boundaries, the production of phenomena which are material-cultural intra-actions. That is, our constructed knowledge has real material consequences" (Barad 1996, p. 183).

Barad draws inspiration from Niels Bohr's interpretation of two classic experiments in physics on the properties of light. One experiment demonstrated that light exists as a wave, while another setup showed light as particles. Bohr argued that light is not some abstract, independent entity with inherent characteristics. Rather, the phenomenon of light interacts with the apparatus. The two experimental apparatuses allow the physicists to perform different agential cuts, which create different material resolutions. In other words, when people build artefacts (e.g., apparatuses, in Bohr's case) they create order in the entanglement. They constitute their world. The agential cut takes place as we couple together the artefact and enact it in practice. You change the artefact and, with it, you change the world you enact and experience. In Barad's words, "the measurement of unambiguously defined quantities is possible through the introduction of a constructed cut which serves to define 'object' and 'agencies of observations' in a particular context" (Barad 1996, p. 171). Following a similar line of thinking, Suchman (2007) argues that it takes boundary work, framing, and cutting to delineate discrete units of artefacts, people, and performances. Such bounding and cutting, joining and separating are the everyday business of doctors, nurses, designers, and social scientists alike.

2.3.4 Four Basic Assumptions from Sociomateriality

Four basic assumptions from sociomateriality are particularly important in our sociomaterial-design approach. *First*, when we study practice, we study a world that is already sliced and diced by practitioners' agential cuts into a gallery of artefacts, doings, and discourses. In order to perform, practitioners bind the world into actionable bundles. So, when we as designers enter a practice, we face bundles of bits and pieces nicely bound and cut for action by practitioners.

Second, we cannot regard these bundles of artefacts, doings, and discourses as *pre-given* and timeless entities. "Boundaries are not fixed" (Barad 1996, p. 180). Each and every artefact is produced and reproduced through our own and others' agential cuts with social and historical consequences. Knorr-Cetina (1997) and Suchman (2007) discuss these as configurations and re-configurations, a process that constantly reworks the sociomaterial arrangements through people's ongoing practices.

Third, the artefacts we enact are always part of *smaller and larger entanglements* (Barad 2003). For instance, we can approach the sociomaterial practices associated with the medical record in a clinic as one entity. Simultaneously, we could also break the medical record apart by focusing solely on the sociomaterial practices associated with one single document in the record. It all depends on the agential cuts we as researchers or designers perform. Each agential cut we create forms the boundaries for the nexus of doings, materialities, and discourses that we study.

Finally, when we submit to the notion that we cannot tease apart the social and the material, nor pinpoint universal properties, it allows us the freedom to perform multiple agential cuts operating at matching times and places. Without pre-determined boundaries of what makes the artefacts, much analytical work is required to distinguish the relations relevant for the purpose of design. Creating these distinctions is about creating and examining the dynamic boundaries that make the entities we design for. Boundaries are not our enemies; instead, they are necessary for making meaning. Thus, a critical part of our work as sociomaterial-designers is to seek out the dynamic boundaries by identifying existing boundaries through the process of boundary making.

2.4   Design

Before we start discussing sociomaterial-design, we need to make another stop and visit current design research in order to understand its foundations and interests, in general and for healthcare practices in particular. This will ensure that these interests are taken seriously in the sociomaterial-design approach. The purpose of this chapter is not to provide a complete overview of all design research (if such a complete overview is even possible), but instead to provide a condensed categorization of research on design in healthcare from various disciplinary perspectives. For some readers (Ada) this might be common knowledge and if so, please skip the chapter. However, for others (Alan) this section might offer new insights into the disciplinary interests of design (Fig. 2.3).

It is crucial to note that design practice is not a distinctly different activity from that of design research. In disciplines such as CSCW, CHI, or PD, there are no separations between what constitute research activities and what constitute design activities, since these are tightly coupled. When design researchers engage in research activities, they design and vice versa. Activities such as experimentation, empirical investigation, modelling, and theory building are frequently done in concert with design practices such as identifying needs, forming new objects, and crafting new practices (Dourish and Bell 2011). Design is the response to experiences in practice by "creating novel artefacts to facilitate our activities and enrich our experiences" (Carrol 1987, p. 19). Design constitutes the "practice of inventing, creating, and implementing (technical) artefacts that depends upon, integrates, and transforms heterogeneous and uncertain domains of knowledge" (Bergman et al. 2007, p. 547). Design research strives to change and ultimately improve practice through the design of artefacts. The fundamental interest of design research is to carve out opportunities for new performances, which can come to life through concrete artefacts. It does so by starting with the complexity of practical circumstances but ultimately

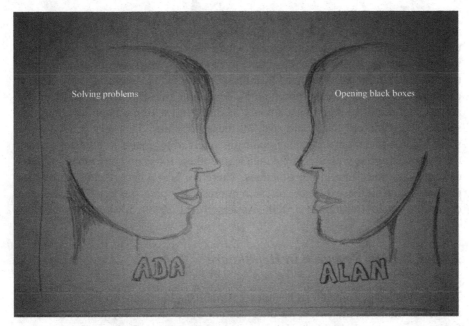

Fig. 2.3 Solving problems or opening black boxes

striving for the design of particular artefacts. Without synthesizing everyday activities into formal representations that reduce the intricacies of the IT landscape, it becomes difficult to develop IT interventions (Adomavicius et al. 2008) and design new artefacts. The research contributions of design research thus, broadly speaking, fall into three main categories: the practical use and understanding of design practices; the result of the design, as in the artefact; and how the design becomes part of the organization relevant for the design, also referred to as design-in-use.

> [T]he origin of design is in involved practical use and understanding, not detached reflection, and design is seen as an interaction between understanding and creativity. (Pelle Ehn 1993 qouted in Robertson and Simonsen 2013, p. 8)

Design is definitely not a routine activity, but requires time, engagement, and creativity, as well as the ability to transform wild ideas to concrete constructions of the artefacts in question. While everyone can get crazy ideas, it is the difficult job of the designer to transform these into realistic manifestations that can facilitate intervention in practice. A major challenge in this process is in moving from description of current situations in the world towards future scenarios after the intervention, especially since the empirical descriptions are often ethnographic descriptions (Blomberg et al. 1993) that are supposed to drive the design reasoning, but are "incomplete, inaccurate, or irrelevant" (Carrol 1987, p. 19). Ethnographic descriptions are not *a priori* directed at design, and it takes time, effort, and interdisciplinary competence to move from complex descriptions of the world into concrete discussions about data structures, interfaces, and system architectures. As Dourish writes:

"despite our best intentions, field studies and design activities often sit uncomfortable together" (Dourish 2004, p. 155). Design research, at least in a theoretical utopia, is in this way a creative activity where the researcher engages with a field with the aim of creating a technical intervention, which then can be tried in practice. In research practice, studying healthcare work practices, transforming empirical observations into design opportunities, designing artefacts, and then testing the artefacts all require a significant amount of time, and within one project there are seldom the resources that could span all these activities. This means that, while some studies focus on the ethnographically interesting analysis, others focus on the design activities with users, and then again others focus on constructing technical artefacts to test in real-life situations. There are also what are called off-cause projects, when all these different research interests and practices come together and create one whole (Bardram et al. 2006; Andersen et al. 2009), however they are rare.

2.4.1   Design Research in Healthcare

Technology design research on healthcare is published in many diverse venues that altogether make up the *corpus* of the research. Some of the key journal and conference venues include *Medical Informatics, Information Systems, Participatory Design, Computer Human Interaction*, and *Computer Supported Cooperative Work*. Whereas these fields each have their own interests, agendas, and lines of research, they together form the majority of research on technology design for healthcare practices. Our intention here is not to create a complete review of all this literature.[1] Rather, our intention is to point to some of the types or categories of design research for healthcare in order to create a common ground for the kind of work that researchers like Ada conduct.

Broadly speaking, there are three different types for design research for healthcare: *technology-centred, organizational-centred*, or *method-centred*. Briefly, technology-centred research makes the design of the digital systems supporting healthcare practice the main focus; organizational-centred research makes the design within the healthcare organizations the main focus: and, finally, method-centred research makes the design methods the main focus—for instance, as in how to engage participants (medical professionals, as well as patients) within the design of both technology and organization. While each of these particular types of research is often published in particular venues (for example, design methods research is often published at conferences such as PDC and NordiCHI), it is important to note that researchers move between the fields, conferences, and journals. Also, since healthcare technologies are part of an interdisciplinary field (Chiasson et al. 2007), this means that the clear boundaries we make between fields are dispersed within

---

[1] For a great extensive overview of design research in healthcare see Fitzpatrick, G. and G. Ellingsen (2013). "A review of 25 years of CSCW research in Healthcare: Contributions, Challenges and future agendas." Computer Supported Cooperative Work (CSCW): An International Journal 22: 609–665.

these technologies—and research findings in this area are typically found explicitly in special issues (Aarts et al. 2010; Bansler and Kensing 2010; Reddy et al. 2011; Bjørn and Kensing 2013).

Technology-centred design research is an endeavor in which the focus is on the design of the technical artefact—the technical system. In many cases, these studies start off with collaborations between design researchers and medical professionals with an interest in technology. This might include situations where medical doctors want to improve the practices of decision making (Frykholm and Groth 2011), or evaluate the implementation of a particular technology within a practice (Tang and Carpendale 2008; Zhou et al. 2012). The technologies can be particular artefacts, such as electronic patient records (Hertzum and Simonsen 2008), or more complex systems, such as hospital information systems (Aarts et al. 2007; Ellingsen et al. 2013), document handling systems (Boulus and Bjørn 2008), electronic medical record systems (Johannesen et al. 2013), or telemedicine technologies (Andersen et al. 2010). Similar to technology-centred research, this type of research shares an interest in the organizational, economic, social, and clinical impact of information systems in healthcare; however, it is important to note that for studies within this particular research area the technical artefact is the main focus. It is also important to mention that the system focus does not make the field particularly design-oriented, since the focus is more on how the technical system is implemented and impacts the medical practice. The general aim of healthcare informatics is to develop healthcare practices with technology, and the basic assumption is that technology will have a direct impact on the practices, thus concepts such as "supports" and "causes" are frequently used (see e.g. Hertzum and Simonsen 2008). The ontological understanding of the broad category of designing healthcare systems supporting medical practice is thus very different from the ontological understanding of socio-materiality. This does not mean that venues for technology-centred design research, such as healthcare informatics conferences and journals, are not open to the social organization of work and how it impacts the medical practice—they clearly are (e.g. Berg 2001). But our point is that while there is an interest in the larger social issues around technical systems, it is the technical system that always becomes the focal point.

Organizational-centred design research is typically published under the very large umbrella of information systems research. However, here we are not interested in all information system research, but only the part which concerns the design of healthcare systems (Chiasson et al. 2007). The field of information systems does not produce purely technical papers (see for an example of this, the scope of *Information System Journal*), but insists on viewing technologies according to the perspectives of implementation, development, strategy, management, or policy (see for an example, the scope of *European Journal of Information Systems*). This means that this type of healthcare research is different at its core from the technological-centred research by having the social organization of work as the focal point (e.g. Chiasson and Davidson 2004). This clear focus on the social organization has caused the IT artefact to disappear in information system research (Orlikowski and Iacono 2001). Thus, design healthcare research is a less prevalent category of information systems research that still preserves the interest in the IT artefact. Comparing the technology-centred healthcare design research with the organizational-centred healthcare design research, we might say that the former has a tendency to privilege the IT artefact; whereas, the latter might have the opposite tendency, namely to privilege the social organization of work. The social organization of healthcare work includes topics on standardization and re-configuration (Hanseth et al. 2006; Bjørn et al. 2009), as well as professional sense-making (Jensen and Aanestad 2007).

Method-centred design research is research where making the agenda on design practices and activities is the focal point (Simonsen and Robertsen 2013). In many situations method-centred design research for healthcare starts off with the sociotechnical approaches for participatory design, and thus is also founded in the Scandinavian tradition of designing with users (see the previous chapter on socio-technical approaches). This tradition has produced several techniques and methods that were created to ensure user participation (Ehn 1989; Bødker and Buur 2002; Bødker et al. 2004). In this tradition, research on healthcare focuses on helping out patients and medical professionals by creating technologies that enable their work (Hartswood et al. 2002). Such work might focus specifically on facilitating and empowering patients (Andersen 2013), understanding chronic diseases (Chen 2011), or physically challenging patients (Bagalkot and Sokolar 2011; Galliers et al. 2012). Compared to technology-centred research, method-centred research also focuses on the designed artefacts, but *include*s explicit explorations of the practices, techniques, and methods by which artefacts become designed with the participants. Comparing the method-centred perspective with the organizational-centred perspective, we find that the method perspective includes organizational interests, but that such interests focus in most cases on the satisfaction of the workers and the democratic agendas, while the organizational-centred research tends to provide more of a managerial perspective. The political interest in healthcare has largely been in making the invisible work involved in healthcare function (Strauss et al. 1985; Suchman 1995), however such work is seldom published at the method-centred venues. Instead such studies are more likely to be published elsewhere, for example in CSCW publications (for an example see Møller and Bjørn 2011).

2.4.2   Designing for Healthcare: Computer-supported Cooperative Work

There are many links between participatory design and *computer-supported cooperative work* (CSCW) to be found when we explore the design research on healthcare, for example in terms of the political interest (Bjørn and Balka 2007a) and how the basic foundations of designers' work is explored by investigating the assumptions behind technological artefacts (Jensen 2007). However, what makes CSCW unique is the dual interest in studying the basic nature of the collaborative practice with the aim of designing collaborative systems (Schmidt and Bannon 1992). Artefacts supporting cooperative work, such as the work in EDs, can be conceptualized as "runtime abstractions encapsulating and providing coordination services" for the

Fig. 2.4 Timestamp machine located on triage desk in an emergency department

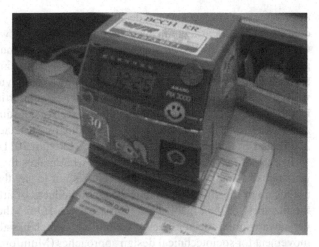

collaborative participants in a given social context (Ricci et al. 2005, p. 191). Artefacts are the concrete physical incarnation of the designer's abstractions of the work that supposedly should be supported. In this way, the physical materiality of the artefact takes a representational role by serving a particular coordinative function in practice (Fig. 2.4). The physical material expression of the artefact "offers cues to other actors as to the intentions of the actor or actors effecting the changes" (Schmidt and Wagner 2004, p. 15).

One key principle in CSCW research is that the material properties of artefacts matter. Numerous studies demonstrate, for instance, how different material properties of paper versus electronic documents all play a part in what shapes the collaborative space (Luff et al. 2000; Sellen and Harper 2002). We also find rich literature discussing how coordinative artefacts, by their physical material properties, are enacted in the complex circumstances of collaborative work arrangements (Bjørn and Rødje 2008). Materiality matters for design. The "design and deployment of new technology should support the functions provided by physical artefacts replaced or disrupted by new technology, and profitable ways for new technology to support collaborative work by embedding ICT into existing infrastructure of physical artefact" (Xiao 2005, p. 26). In other words, when changing the materiality from a tangible physical object into an electronic artefact, the transformations go beyond the immediate functionalities of the old and the new system; Each has to be molded to fit into the collaborative practices and the types of cues they may or may not offer.

Considering the materiality of one coordinative artefact is quite different from understanding a complex work setting with a complex sociomaterial nexus of doings, materialities, and discourses. Yet, given a preoccupation with the design, implementation, and use of coordinative artefacts, many scholars end up studying one system at a time (Xiao et al. 2001; Chiasson and Davidson 2004; Xiao 2005; Hanseth et al. 2006; Boulus and Bjørn 2008; Bjørn et al. 2009). Although these studies are important, they tend to neglect how each of these systems and their materiality function not in isolation, but are part of larger and smaller entanglements. This is not to say that design researchers are not aware of the multiplicity of practice and artefacts. Many design researchers try to capture the multiplicity of coordinative work arrangements, particularly in hospital work (Hanseth et al. 2006; Cho et al. 2008). Moreover, different perspectives on multiplicity have been suggested in design research, such as ecosystems representing the many technologies and relationships that make up the IT landscape (Adomavicius et al. 2008), a patchwork of systems understood as the infrastructure supporting the IS systems within healthcare (Ellingsen and Monteiro 2003), a web of coordinative artefacts (Bardram and Bossen 2005), the multiplicity of coordinative artefacts (Schmidt and Wagner 2004), and artefactual multicity (Bjørn and Hertzum 2011).

In each of these approaches, however, what makes the "artefact"—its boundaries—remains stable and pre-defined. This is not to say that design researchers are not aware of the situatedness and the embodiedness of artefact (Dourish 2004), or the fuzziness of the organization (Ciborra 1996). Quite the contrary: Designers are very aware of the social aspect of technology, which has also been confirmed in the movement for sociotechnical design approaches (Mumford 2006). One key element of the socio-technical research stream is that the interconnections are understood as emergent and thus not determining, and this stream of research adopts a "processual logic where interactions and outcomes are seen to be mutually dependent, integrative, and co-evolving over time" (Orlikowski and Scott 2008, p. 446). Nevertheless, in the socio-technical design agenda, the boundaries for what makes the artefact are pre-determined. An artefact is an artefact with stable boundaries—and it is easy to point to the boundaries (Fig. 2.5).

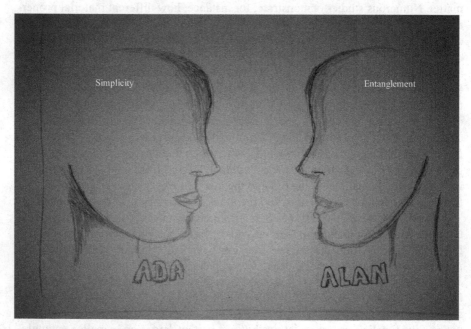

Fig. 2.5 Simplicity and entanglement

2.5 Point of Departure for Sociomaterial-design

If we are to create a sociomaterial-design approach, we have to articulate an analytical approach that pays keen attention to artefacts, old and new, existing in a nexus of doings, materialities, and discourses, but without regarding the boundaries of the artefacts as pre-given. We need an analytical strategy that helps us untangle what appears as given artefacts with solid boundaries but opens up as artefacts with dynamic boundaries.

The analytical strategy refers to how Ada and Alan together can conduct research; that is the *research practices*, by which the researchers together can approach the healthcare practice and start to work. Now, the way we will demonstrate the analytical strategy and practical accomplishment of sociomaterial-design is through our empirical cases; however, before we dive into all the empirical complexities we encountered while engaging ourselves in the sociomaterial practices in EDs, we want to set the scaffold for our departure into sociomaterial-design, and thus create the starting point for how to engage with sociomaterial-design.

Healthcare practice is a professional practice in which participants constantly and dynamically engage with artefacts, technologies, people, and processes. Healthcare practice is also a sociomaterial practice in which technologies, organizational processes, people, and artefacts are continually entangled and not easily taken apart. Using the words of Barad (Barad 2003), sociomaterial-designers meet a world sliced and diced by agential cuts created by the practitioners: In this case, the doctors and nurses who, to perform their work, have to bundle their world into dynamic entities of objects and activities. Exploring practice thus entails figuring out the agential cuts of the practitioners. There are uncountable possible variations as to how these agential cuts are made by the practitioners, and it is not easy to figure out which to explore. This multiplicity of agential cuts is what researchers such as Alan really appreciate and find fascinating. It is the opening onto and subsequent following of a different path that continuously increases the nuanced and increasing complex world of healthcare practices. However, if we are to take into account our *objective*, namely to engage Alan in collaboration with Ada and thus engage both of them with design *without* reducing the complex important intra-actions between the enactment in the sociomaterial practices in the healthcare practice, we need to *reconfigure* the sociomaterial agenda towards the design agenda of Ada. Ada designs artefacts and regardless of whether she engages with design practices centred on technologies, organizations, or methods, the artefact is what is most immediately significant. Design interventions are basically about artefacs and thus, if we are to sensitize the sociomaterial agenda toward design, the point of departure must be the artefact. So the artefact becomes our significant centre for sociomaterial-design, however we also need to *bend* design towards the sociomaterial agenda. It is therefore not only the sociomaterial agenda that gets reconfigured; the design agenda also needs to be reconfigured, if we are to create the new entity of sociomaterial-design. This bending involves an ontological change, where the boundaries and borders that make the artefacts are not pre-determined, but instead dynamic and flexible. But what does this mean?

2.5.1   From Agential Cuts to Bounding Practices

Doctors and nurses will happily point you to their favorite artefacts or explain their shortcomings. It might be possible to point at a physical and material artefact with your finger, and when you take the object in your hand you can touch the borders around the artefact. The borders for what makes the artefact are immediately physical and tangible and by brushing your hand over the surface and you can feel its properties. However, it is important to note that this connection through touch along the surface of the artefact is *not* what constitutes the sociomaterial boundaries of the artefact. Sure artefacts in most cases appear as tangible and physical entities, with physical boundaries that you can touch and feel. But, these boundaries are not the boundaries for the sociomaterial artefact, and without expanding the perspective on what makes the boundaries of the artefact to include the dynamic bounding practices which healthcare professionals create when enacting the artefact, you cannot engage with the sociomaterial practices and thus will have a reduced perspective of what makes the space for design. The sociomaterial-designer needs to expand her perspective and sensitivity towards the sociomaterial practices by which the healthcare professionals enact the artefacts we want to innovate. However to do this we need to expand our vocabulary and our sensitivity as researchers.

Much has been inspired by Barad's concept of agential cuts, wherein she makes the experimental apparatus part of the observed matter in Niels Bohr's experiment on the properties of light, and we take a similar approach here. When healthcare professionals enact in practice each artefact they engage with is constitutive of the practices. This means that the boundaries of what make the artefact are dynamically created and co-created during the actual practices. In other words, when people act in practice they bind together artefact in the sociomaterial practices. We refer to this process as bounding practices. *Bounding practices* are the practices wherein people simultaneously bind together artefacts and human activities, while creating boundaries for what is inside and what becomes outside of the artefact. To provide an example, when a nurse picks up a clipboard and places it on a chart rack, he simultaneously binds together the clipboard-chartrack, while he creates the boundaries for what makes the artefact [clipboard-chartrack]. Bounding practices are about *binding-together while* [*bracketing out*] sociomaterial artefacts in a temporal manner, since the boundaries for what make the sociomaterial artefact are constantly changing as the artefact emerges as part of different sociomaterial practices.

2.5.2   What Is a Boundary?

With the focus on bounding practices it is important that we also reflect upon what makes a boundary? Boundaries have been a topic for various type of research and been investigated in terms of "boundary objects" (Star and Griesemer 1989), "boundary infrastructures" (Bowker and Star 2002), "boundary organizations" (Guston), and "boundary work" (Gieryn). We will now visit each of these conceptualizations of boundaries and apply these to advance our conceptualization of boundaries as it generally applies to our conceptual understanding of bounding practices. *Boundary objects* are both plastic enough to adapt to local practices across diverse intersecting social worlds, yet robust enough to maintain a common identity (Star and Griesemer 1989). Thus, the "boundary" term in the conceptual understanding of boundary objects emphasizes the how the object remains the same while travelling across the boundaries of various social worlds. The boundary becomes the intersection between social worlds. Based upon the work on "boundary objects," Bowker and Star (2002) introduce *boundary infrastructures*, which concerns the categorical work involving the multiple complex sets of relations at its centre rather than focusing on the singular object. The concept of "boundary" in this understanding refers to boundaries between highly complex sets of diverse communities, wherein classification within boundary infrastructures serves as a powerful tool and technology for making such community interact. *Boundary organizations* emerge from research on the intersections between the two large communities of politics and science (Guston 2001), and a boundary organization attempts to provide opportunity and incentives for the creation and use of boundary objects across the two different social worlds of politics and science by involving participations from all sides the boundary through distinct lines of accountability for each party (Guston 2001, p. 400). The focus is thus to highlight practices by which the boundary organization can speak differently to different audiences.

Boundary object, boundary infrastructure, and boundary organizations all refer to the "boundary" as the intersection between diverse heterogeneous social entities (e.g., social worlds, communities, or organizations). Our concept of boundary is of a different nature. Boundaries in sociomaterial-design are the constantly changing results emerging from the enactment of artefacts within the collaborative practice—a practice that we refer to as bounding practice. However, we still need to create a closer definition of what a boundary is. For this reason, our last stop in our analysis of literature is *boundary work* (Fig. 2.6).

Boundary work refers to the work by which scientists create the boundary between what is science and what is none-science (Gieryn 1983). Interestingly, the

Fig. 2.6 Researcher inside the emergency department

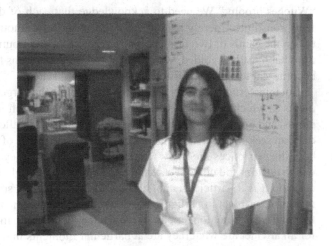

boundary work done by scientists is not concerned with how scientists try to cross the boundary and make their work accessible to people outside the research community. Instead, boundary work is the work by which scientists construct the boundary between what is inside and what is outside. This construction of the boundary is done for different reasons at different times, and scientists apply different strategies in their boundary making. What the concept of boundary work points to is the malleable dynamic entity that makes a boundary, and how such boundaries do not exist *a priori*, but instead changes over time. Our conceptualization of bounding practices very much resembles boundary work by replying on the similar definition of a *boundary* as something which is "ambiguous, flexible, historical changing, contextually variable, internally inconsistent, and sometime disputed" (Gieryn 1983, p. 792). However, where boundary work emphasis the creation and making of particular communities (such as scientific communities) from a rhetorical perspective, *our* bounding practices concerns the creation of the sociomaterial properties which makes the collaborative artefacts within concrete professional work practices.

2.5.3 *Bounding Practices as Analytical Strategy*

When Ada and Alan engage in common research endeavors of sociomaterial-design, their shared immediate interest is therefore the *bounding practices* they encounter when entering the ED. However, it is important to note that we, as sociomaterial-designers, meet this new research agenda not as a blank slate but populated by our own bounding practice—how we think the world is bound and bracketed together. Therefore, sociomaterial-design is a practice wherein the Ada and Alan re-configure their own bounding practices toward the experienced bounding practices of the healthcare practitioners.

Sociomaterial-designers cannot simply map the artefacts and practices already bound and bracketed together for them by the practitioners. Invoking Haraway's image of cat's cradle (Haraway 1994), we argue that practitioners have a tendency to present particularly prominent or favored patterns, be it "Jacob's ladder" or "Witches broom." We need to acknowledge that each of these sociomaterial artefacts constitutes merely a stopping point in the continuous passing of strings between the hands of two or more participants. Existing bounding practices present a trap that must be avoided. We must not rest on the notions that the boundaries have become stable, since stability is only a temporal state.

Sociomaterial-designers can do so by tracing the larger and smaller entanglements in which prominent bounding practices nest. Each nexus of doings, materialities, and discourses can be disassembled to reveal smaller bounding practices, or one can seek to understand the larger bounding practices of which it is a part. These bounding practices are more than analytical moves. They change the world upon which doctors and nurses act. As in Niels Bohr's case, light *is* a wave in one agential cut, and it *is* a particle in another (Barad 2003). In this same way, each bounding makes the artefact in particular way, and places the boundaries for what is the artefact and what is not longer part of the artefact, which also means that the boundaries for an artefact are what they are at particular moments in time.

Tracking larger and smaller entanglements associated with prominent bounding practices involves the bounding and rebounding of artefacts, locations, and people's movements. After having mapped the artefacts associated with prominent bounding practices, the sociomaterial-designer takes a step back and starts experimenting with different ways to bind and bundle artefacts, locations, and people's movements. By unfolding sociomaterial practices we found that by "cutting" the practice up in different analytical distinctions, first bounding artefacts with other artefacts, then bounding artefacts with the different locations they travel to, and then finally bounding artefacts and people's movements, the sociomateriality of the practices becomes apparent and available to us as sociomaterial-designers, thus we can start to create reflective innovations within the practice.

We argue that this progressive analytical approach will reveal less prominent bounding practices performed by practitioners and lead to a better understanding of what "things" are and how things get done in the particular setting. Likewise, it becomes a tool for sociomaterial-designers to envision new bounding practices associated with new artefacts and how they will nest into the larger and smaller entanglements already in place. Like a game of cat's cradle, the sociomaterial designer traces how the strings move from hand to hand, revealing at each turn a new nexus; then she *additionally* traces the movement of the yarn and the multiple ways it is bound, not only as the pattern string figures, but as the bundle of yarn which comes into being between the appealing patterns. We no longer have to seek only either pre-given artefacts or an entangled mess, we look at each of these in relation to each other.

This marks our point of departure from our academic discussions and into discussions of the healthcare practices within EDs (Fig. 2.7).

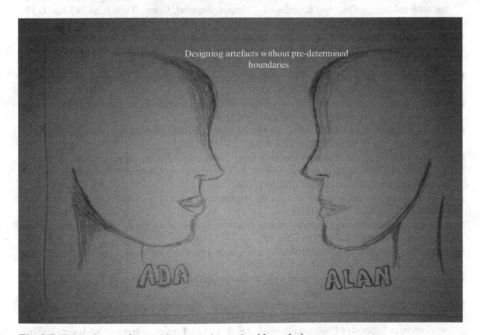

Designing artefacts without pre-determined boundaries

ADA   ALAN

Fig. 2.7 Designing artefacts without pre-determined boundaries

References

Aarts, J., Ash, J., et al.: Extending the understanding of computerized physician order entry: implications for professional collaboration, workflow and quality of care. Int. J. Med. Inform. **76**, 4–13 (2007)

Aarts, J., Callen, J., et al.: Information technology in health care: socio-technical approaches. Int. J. Med. Inform. **79**(6), 389–390 (2010)

Adomavicius, G., Bockstedt, J., et al.: Making sense of technology trends in the information technology landscape: a design science approach. MIS Q. **32**(4), 779–809 (2008)

Akrich, M., Latour, B.: A summary of a convenient Vocabulary for the semiotics of human and nonhuman assemblies. In: Bijker, W., Law, J. (eds.) Shaping Technology Building Society. Studies in Sociotechnical Change. MIT Press, Cambridge (1992)

Andersen, T.: Medication Management in the Making: On Ethnography-design Relations. Computer Supported Cooperative Work, pp. 1103–1112. ACM, San Antonio (2013)

Andersen, N.E., Kensing, F., et al.: Professionel Systemudvikling: Erfaringer, Muligheder og Handling. Teknisk Forlag A/S, Århus (1986)

Andersen, T., Bansler, J., et al.: Co-constructing IT and healthcare. Poster Paper Presented at European Conference Computer Supported Cooperative Work (ECSCW). Vienna, Austria (2009)

Andersen, T., Bjørn, P., et al.: Designing for collaborative interpretation in telemonitoring: re-introducing patients as diagnostic agents. Int. J. Med. Inform. (2010). doi:10.1016/j.ijmedinf.2010.09.010

Bagalkot, N., Sokolar, T.: MyReDiary: co-designing for collaborative articulation in physical rehabilitation. European Conference of Computer Supported Cooperative work (ECSCW), pp. 121–132. Springer, Århus (2011)

Bannon, L., Bødker, S.: Constructing common information spaces. Fifth European Conference on Computer Supported Cooperative Work, Kluwer Academic Publisher (1997)

Bannon, L., Bjørn, P., et al.: Building a socially embedded future internet. http://fisa.future-internet.eu/images/f/ff/VolkerWulf_Socially_Embedded_Computing.pdf (2012). Accessed December 2013

Bansler, J., Kensing, F.: Information infrastructure for health care: connecting practices across institutional and professional boundaries. Comput. Support. Coop. Work (CSCW) Int. J. **19**, 519–520 (2010)

Barad, K.: Meeting the universe halfway: realism and social constructivism without contradiction. In: Nelson, L.H., Nelson, J. (eds.) Feminism, Science, and the Philosophy of Science, pp. 161–194. Kluwer Academic Publishers, London (1996)

Barad, K.: Posthumanist performativity: toward an understanding of how matter comes to matter. Signs: J. Women Cult. Soc. **28**(3), 801–831 (2003)

Barad, K.: Meeting the Universe Halfway: Quantum Physics and the Entanglement of Matter and Meaning. Duke University Press, Durham (2007)

Bardram, J., Bossen, C.: Mobility work: the spatial dimension of collaboration at a hospital. Comput. Support. Coop. Work (CSCW) Int. J. **14**, 131–160 (2005)

Bardram, J., Hansen, T., et al.: AwareMedia: a shared interactive display supporting social, temporal, and spatial awareness in surgery. CSCW'06 Conference on Computer Supported Cooperative Work, Banff, Alberta, Canada, ACM (2006)

Berg, M.: Patient care information systems and health care work: a sociotehcnical approach. Int. J. Med. Inform. **55**, 87–101 (1999)

Berg, M.: Implementing information systems in healthcare organizations: myths and challenges. Int. J. Med. Inform. **64**, 143–156 (2001)

Bergman, M., Lyytinen, K., et al.: Boundary objects in design: an ecological view of design artefacts. J. Assoc. Inf. Syst. **8**(11), 546–568 (2007)

Bjørn, P.: Bounding practice: how people act in sociomaterial practices. Scand. J. Inf. Syst. **24**(2), 97–104 (2012)

Bjørn, P., Balka, E.: Health care categories have politics too: unpacking the managerial agendas of electronic triage systems. ECSCW 2007: Proceedings of the Tenth European Conference on Computer Supported Cooperative Work, pp. 371–390, Limerick, Ireland, Springer (2007a)

Bjørn, P., Balka, E.: Technology transforms the space for knowledge acquisition. ED-media, World Conference on Educational Multimedia, Hybermedia and Telecommunication, Vancouver, Canada, ACM (2007b)

Bjørn, P., Hertzum, M.: Artefactual multiplicity: a study of emergency-department whiteboards. Comput. Support. Coop. Work (CSCW) Int. J. **20**(1), 93 (2011)

Bjørn, P., Kensing, F.: Special issue on information infrastructures for healthcare: the global and local relation. Int. J. Med. Inform. **82**, 281–282 (2013)

Bjørn, P., Markussen, R.: Cyborg heart: the affective apparatus of bodily production of ICD patients. Sci. Technol. Stud. **26**(2) (2013)

Bjørn, P., Rødje, K.: Triage drift: a workplace study in a pediatric emergency department. Comput. Support. Coop. Work (CSCW) Int. J. **17**(4), 395–419 (2008)

Bjørn, P., Burgoyne, S., et al.: Boundary factors and contextual contingencies: configuring electronic templates for health care professionals. Eur. J. Inf. Syst. **18**, 428–441 (2009)

Blomberg, J., Karasti, H.: Reflections on 25 years or ethnography in CSCW. Comput. Support. Coop. Work (CSCW) Int. J. **22**, 373–423 (2013)

Blomberg, J., Giacomi, J., et al.: Ethnographic field methods and their relation to design. In: Schuler, D., Namioka, A. (eds.) Participatory Design: Principles and Practices, pp. 123–155. Lawrence Erlbaum Associates Publisher, London (1993)

Bødker, S., Buur, J.: The design collaboratorium—a place for usability design. ACM Trans. Comput. Hum. Interact. **9**(2), 152–169 (2002)

Bødker, S., Ehn, P., et al.: Co-operative Design—perspectives on 20 years with 'the Scandinavian IT Design Model'. Kungl Tekniska Hogskolan, Stockholm (2000)

Bødker, K., Kensing, F., et al.: Participatory IT design: Designing for Business and Workplace Realities. MIT Press, Cambridge (2004)

Boulus, N., Bjørn, P.: A cross-case analysis of technology-in-use practices: EPR-adaptation in Canada and Norway. Int. J. Med. Inform. **79**(6), 97–108 (2008)

Bowker, G.C., Star, S.L.: Sorting Things Out: Classification and Its Consequences. MIT Press, Cambridge (2002)

Bratteteig, T., Verne, G.: Conditions for autonomy in the information society: disentangling as a public service. Scand. J. Inf. Syst. **24**(2), 51–78 (2012)

Carlsson, J., Ehn, P., et al.: Planning and control from the perspective of labour: a short presentation of the Demos project. Account. Organ. Soc. **3**(3/4), 249–260 (1978)

Carrol, J.: Interfacing Thought: Cognitive Aspects of Human-computer Interaction. MIT Press, Cambridge (1987)

Cecez-Kecmanovic, D., Galliers, B., Henfridsson, O., Newell, S., and Vidgen, R. Call for papers: MISQ special issue on Sociomateriality of information systems and organizing. MIS Quarterly: http://www.misq.org/skin/frontend/default/misq/pdf/CurrentCalls/SI_Sociomateriality.pdf (2011)

Checkland, P., Holwell, S.: Information, Systems and Information Systems—Making Sense of the Field. Wiley, Chichester (1998)

Chen, Y.: Health information use in chronic care cycles. Computer Supported Cooperative Work, pp. 485–488. ACM, China (2011)

Chiasson, M., Davidson, E.: Pushing the contextual envelope: developing and diffusing IS theory for health information system research. Inf. Organ. **14**, 155–188 (2004)

Chiasson, M., Davidson, E.: On Being Relevant to the Future of IS Practice. AMCIS, San Fransisco, AIS (2009)

Chiasson, M., Reddy, M., et al.: Expanding multi-disciplinary approaches to healthcare information technologies: what does information system offer medical informatics? Int. J. Med. Inform. **76S**, 589–597 (2007)

Cho, S., Mathiassen, L., et al.: Contextual dynamics during health information systems implementation: an event-based actor-network approach. Eur. J. Inf. Syst. **17**, 614–630 (2008)

Ciborra, C.: The platform organization: recombining strategies, structures, and surprises. Organ. Sci. **7**(2), 103–118 (1996)

Dourish, P.: Where the Action Is: The Foundations of Embodied Interaction. MIT Press, Cambrigde, London (2004)

Dourish, P., Bell, G.: Divining a Digital Future: Mess and Mythology in Ubiquitous Computing. MIT Press, London (2011)

Dreyfus, H.: Intuitive, deliberative and calculative models of expert performance. In: Zsambok, C., Klein, G. (eds.) Naturalistic Decision Making, pp. 17–28. Lawrence Erlbaum Associates, Mahwah (1997)

Ehn, P.: The art and science of designing computer artefacts. Scand. J. Inf. Syst. **1**, 21–42 (1989)

Ellingsen, G., Monteiro, E.: A patchwork planet integration and cooperation in hospitals. Comput. Support. Coop. Work (CSCW) Int. J. **12**(1), 71–95 (2003)

Ellingsen, G., Monteriro, E., et al.: Integration as interdependent workaround. Int. J. Med. Inform. **82**, 161–169 (2013)

Faraj, S., Azad, B.: The materiality of technology: an affordance perspective. In: Leonardi, P., Nardi, B., Kallinikos, J. (eds.) Materiality and Organizing: Social Interaction in a Technological World, pp. 237–258. Oxford University Press (2012)

Fitzpatrick, G., Ellingsen, G.: A review of 25 years of CSCW research in healthcare: contributions, challenges and future agendas. Comput. Support. Coop. Work (CSCW) Int. J. **22**, 609–665 (2013)

Flores, F., Graves, M., et al.: Computer systems and the design of organizational interaction. ACM Trans. Off. Inf. Syst. **6**(2), 153–172 (1988)

Frykholm, O., Groth, K.: References to personal experiences and scientific evidence during medical multi-disciplinary team meetings. Behav. Inf. Technol. **30**(4), 455–466 (2011)

Galliers, J., Wilson, S., et al.: Words are not Enough: Empowering People with Aphasia in the Design Process. Participatory Design (PDC). ACM, Roskilde (2012)

Gaskin, J., Berente, N., et al.: Towards generalizable sociomaterial inquiry: a computational approach for zooming in and out of sociomaterial routines. MIS Q. **38**(3) 849–871 (2013)

Gieryn, T.: Boundary-work and demarcation of science from non-science: strains and interests in professional ideologies of scientists. Am. Sociol. Rev. **48**(6), 781–795 (1983)

Grudin, J.: CSCW'88: Report on the conference & review of the proceedings. SIGCHI Bull. **20**(4), 80–84 (1988)

Grudin, J., Grinter, R.: Ethnography and design. Comput. Support. Coop. Work (CSCW) Int. J. **3**, 55–59 (1995)

Guston, D.: Boundary organizations in environmental policy and science: an introduction. Sci. Technol. Hum. Values. **26**(4: Special issue), 399–408 (2001)

Hammer, M.: Reengineering work: don't automate, obliterate. Harward Bus. Rev. **68**(4), July–August, 104–112 (1990)

Hanseth, O., Jacussi, E., et al.: Reflexive standardization: side-effects and complexity in standard making. MIS Q. **30**(Special issue on Standard Making), 563–581 (2006)

Haraway, D.: Reading the National Geographic on Primates. Tape number 126. http://www.egs.edu/faculty/donna-haraway/videos/reading-the-national-geographic-on-primates/ (1987). Accessed December 2013

Haraway, D.: A manifesto for cyborgs: science, technology, and socialist feminism in the 1980s. In: Nicholson, L. (ed.) Feminism/Postmodernisme. Routlegde, New York (1990)

Haraway, D.: Simians, Cyborgs and Women: The Reinvention of Nature. Free Associations Books, London (1991)

Haraway, D.: A game of cat's cradle: Science studies, feminist theory, cultural studies. Configurations **2**(1), 59–71 (1994)

Hartswood, M., Procter, R., et al.: Co-realization: Towards a principled synthesis of ethnomethodology and participatory design. Scand. J. Inf. Syst. **14**(2), 9–30 (2002)

Hertzum, M., Simonsen, J.: Positive effects of electronic patient records on three clinical activities. Int. J. Med. Inform. **77**(12), 809–817 (2008)

Jensen, C.B.: Sorting attachments: usefulness of STS in healthcare practice and policy. Sci. Cult. **16**(3), 237–251 (2007)

Jensen, T.B., Aanestad, M.: How healthcare professionals 'make sense' of an electronic patient record adoption. Inf. Syst. Manage. **24**(1), 29–42 (2007)

Johannesen, L.K., Obstfelder, A., et al.: Scaling of an information system in a public healthcare market—Infrastructuring from the vendor's perspective. Int. J. Med. Inform. **82**, 180–188 (2013)

Jones, M.: A matter of life and death: Exploring conceptualizations of sociomateriality in the context of critical care. MIS Q. **38**(3), 895–925 (2013)

Kallinikos, J., Asltonen, A., et al.: The ambivalent ontology of digital artefacts. MIS Q. **37**(2), 357–370 (2013)

Kaptelinin, V., Bannon, L.: Interaction design beyond the product: creating technology-enhanced activity spaces. Hum. Comput. Interact. **27**(3), 277–309 (2012)

Kautz, K., Jensen, T.: Debating sociomateriality: entanglements, imbrications, disentangling, and agential cuts. Scand. J. Inf. Syst. **24**(2), 89–96 (2012)

Kensing, F., Simonsen, J., et al.: MUST: a method for participatory design. Hum. Comput. Interact. **13**(2), 167–198 (2009)

Knorr Cetina, K.: Sociality with objects: social relations in postsocial knowledge societies. Theory Cult. Soc. **14**(4), 1–30 (1997)

Krasner, H., Grief, I.: CSCW 86 proceedings of the 1986 ACM conference on Computer-supported cooperative work. CSCW, ACM (1986)

Latour, B.: Science in Action: How to Follow Scientists and Engineers Through Society. Harvard University, Cambridge (1987)

Latour, B.: Reassembling the Social: An Introduction to Actor-Network-Theory, pp. 316. Oxford University Press, Oxford, Sep 2005. ISBN-10: 0199256047; ISBN-13: 9780199256044 1 (2005)

Lave, J., Wenger, E.: Situated Learning Legitimate Peripheral Participation. Cambridge University Press, Cambridge (1991)

Law, J.: After Method: Mess is Social Science Research. Routledge, London (2004)

Leonardi, P.: When flexible routines meet flexible technologies: affordance, constraint, and the imbrication of human and material agencies. MIS Q. **35**(1), 147–167 (2011)

Leonardi, P., Barley, S.: Materiality and change: challenges to building better theory about technology and organizing. Inf. Organ. **18**(3), 159–176 (2008)

Leonardi, P., Barley, S.: What's under construction here? Social action, materiality, and power in constructivist studies of technology and organizing. Acad. Manage. Ann. **4**(1), 1–51 (2010)

Leonardi, P., Nardi, B., Kallinikos, J.: Materiality and Organizing: Social Interaction in a Techno-logical World. Oxford University Press, Oxford (2012)

Luff, P., Hindmarch, J., et al. (eds.): Workplace Studies: Recovering Work Practice and Informing System Design. Cambridge University Press, Cambridge (2000)

Lynch, M.: On making explicit. Comput. Support. Coop. Work (CSCW) Int. J. **3**, 65–68 (1995)

Mathiassen, L.: Reflective system development. Scand. J. Inf. Syst. **10**(1&2), 67–134 (1998)

Mazmanian, M., Cohn, M., Dourish, P.: Dynamic reconfiguration in planetary exploration: a sociomaterial ethnography. MIS Q. **38**(3), 831–848 (2014)

Mol, A.: The Body Multiple: Ontology in Medical Practice. Duke University Press, London (2002)

Møller, N.H., Bjørn, P.: Layers in sorting practices: sorting out patients with potential cancer. Comput. Support. Coop. Work (CSCW) Int. J. **20**, 123–153 (2011)

Mumford, E.: Advice for an action researcher. Inf. Technol. People **14**(1), 12–27 (2001)

Mumford, E.: The story of socio-technical design: reflections on its successes, failures and poten-tial. Inf. Syst. J. **16**, 317–342 (2006)

Orlikowski, W.: Categories: concept, content and context. Comput. Support. Coop. Work (CSCW) Int. J. **3**, 73–78 (1995)

Orlikowski, W.J.: The sociomateriality of organizational life: considering technology in manage-ment research. Camb. J. Econ. **34**, 125–141 (2010)

Orlikowski, W., Iacono, S.: Research commentary: desperately seeking the "IT" in IT research: a call to theorizing the IT artifact. Inf. Syst. Res. **12**(2), 121–134 (2001)

Orlikowski, W., Scott, S.: Sociomateriality: challenging the separation of technology, work, and organization. Acad. Manage. Ann. **2**(1), 433–474 (2008)

Pickering, A.: The Mangle of Practice, Time, Agency and Science. University of Chicago Press, Chicago (1995)

Randall, D., Harper, R., et al.: Fieldwork for Design: Theory and Practice. Springer, London (2007)

Rapoport, R.N.: Three dilemmas in action research. Hum. Relat. **23**(6), 499–513 (1970)

Reckwitz, A.: Toward a theory of social practices: a development in culturalist theorizing. Eur. J. Soc. Theor. **5**, 243–263 (2002)

Reddy, M., Gorman P., et al.: Special issue on supporting collaboration in healthcare settings: the role of informatics. Int. J. Med. Info. **80**(8), 541–543 (2011)

Ricci, A., Viroli M., et al.: Environment-based coordination through coordination artifacts. Lect. Notes. Comput. Sci. **3374**, 190–214 (2005)

Robertson, T., Simonsen, J.: Participatory design: an introduction. Routledge International Handbook of Participatory Design, pp. 1–18. Routledge, London (2013)

Schatzki, T.R., Knorr-Cetina, K., et al. (eds.): The Practice Turn in Contemporary Theory. Routledge, London (2001)

Schmidt, K.: Cooperative Work and Coordinative Practices: Contributions to the Conceptual Foundations Of Computer-Supported Cooperative Work (CSCW). Springer, London (2011)

Schmidt, K., Bannon, L.: Taking CSCW seriously: supporting articulation work. Comput. Support. Coop. Work (CSCW) Int. J. **1**(1–2), 7–40 (1992)

Schmidt, K., Wagner, I.: Ordering systems: coordinative practices and artifacts in architectural design and planning. Comput. Support. Coop. Work **13**, 349–408 (2004)

Sellen, A., Harper, R.: The Myth of the Paperless Office. MIT Press, Cambridge (2002)

Simonsen, J., Robertsen, T.: Routledge International Handbook of Participatory Design. Taylor & Francis Group, Routledge (2013)

Star, S.L., Griesemer, J.: Institutional ecology, translations and boundary objects: amateurs and professionals in Berkeleys museum of Vertebrate zoology, 1907–39. Soc. Stud. Sci. **19**, 387–420 (1989)

Star, S. L., Strauss, A.: Layers of silence, arenas of voice: the ecology of visible and invisible work. Comput. Support. Coop. Work (CSCW) Int. J. **8**, 9–30 (1999)

Strauss, A., Fagerhaugh, S., et al.: Social Organization of Medical Work. The University of Chicago Press, Chicago (1985)

Suchman, L.: Office procedure as practical action: models of work and system design. ACM Trans. Off. Inf. Syst. **1**, 320–328 (1983)

Suchman, L.: Plans and Situated Actions. The Problem of Human Machine Communication. Cambridge University Press, Cambridge (1987)

Suchman, L.: Do categories have politics? The language/action perspective reconsidered. Comput. Support. Coop. Work (CSCW) Int. J. **2**, 177–190 (1994)

Suchman, L.: Making work visible. Commun. ACM. **38**(9), 56–64 (1995)

Suchman, L.: Human-Machine Reconfigurations: Plans and Situated Actions. Cambridge University Press, Cambridge (2007)

Tang, C., Carpendale, S.: Evaluating the deployment of a mobile technology in a hospital ward. Computer Supported Cooperative Work, pp. 205–214. ACM, San Diego (2008)

Trist, E.: The Evolution of Socio-Technical Systems: a Conceptual Framework and an Action Research Program. Ontario Ministry of Labour, Ontario, Canada (1981)

Wenger, E.: Communities of Practice: Learning, Meaning, and Identity. Cambridge University Press, Cambridge (1998)

Wilkie, A., Michael, M.: Expectation and mobilisation: enacting future users. Sci. Technol. Hum. Values **34**(4), 502–522 (2009)

Winner, L.: Do Artifacts have politics? In: Winner, L. (ed.) The Whale and the Reactor: A Search for Limits in an Age of High Technology, pp. 28–40. University of Chicago Press, Chicago (1986)

Winograd, T., Flores, F.: Understanding Computers and Cognition: A New Foundation to System Design. Ablex Publishing Corp, Norwood (1986)

Xiao, Y.: Artifacts and collaborative work in healthcare: methodological theoretical, and technological implications for the tangible. J. Biomed. Info. **38**, 26–33 (2005)

Xiao, Y., Lasome, C., et al.: Cognitive properties of a whiteboard: a case study in a trauma centre. Seventh European Conference on Computer Supported Cooperative work. Bonn, Germany, Kluwer Academic Publisher (2001)

Zhou, X., Zheng K., et al.: Cooperative documentation: the patient problem list as a nexus in electronic health records. Computer Supported Cooperative Work, pp. 911–920. ACM, Seattle (2012)

Part II
Empirical Perspective

Chapter 3
Ethnographic Studies of work in Emergency Departments

The empirical foundation of this book is made up of two longitudinal studies of the work practices and technology design changes in two EDs in North America. In this chapter, we will introduce the empirical cases and the contexts for each of the studies. We decided to introduce the cases as narratives from each of our own personal perspectives as researchers. This will provide the reader insights into how the studies came about and how the sociomaterial-design approach was enacted in practice.

3.1 The Canadian Emergency Department

The empirical study of the work practices within a Canadian ED began in December 2006, when I (Pernille Bjørn) first arrived in Vancouver, Canada, to start on my post-doctoral research at Simon Fraser University. I was hired to conduct post-doctoral research focusing on an electronic triage system that had been implemented 18 months earlier at an ED at a pediatric hospital. The pediatric hospital is a tertiary facility, which means they have the most specialized medical personnel in the entire province and severe cases of children needing medical attention of all kinds are directed to the hospital. The patient demographic of the ED is made up of children younger than 17 years old. The main medical information within the hospital was handled through paper-based archives and processes; however, the hospital wanted to introduce electronic systems to support the work. A first step in the direction of becoming digital in the ED was by implementing an electronic triage system in 2004. This electronic triage system named ETRIAGE (Bullard 2003) had been developed by medical doctors in another province, Alberta. Part of the promised claim of the system was that it facilitated nurses to conduct accurate triage of patients entering the ED. Triage is a key activity in EDs, since it is the process by which patients are sorted based upon the urgency of their chief complaint. In the ED the triage practices were conducted following the Canadian Triage and Acuity Score (CTAS) scheme. CTAS guidelines define that patients are sorted based on a five-point scale, where CTAS level 1 is the highest urgency requiring immediate treatment and CTAS level 5 is basically not sick. The CTAS guidelines also stipulate particular assessment

© Springer International Publishing Switzerland 2014   47
P. Bjørn, C. Østerlund, *Sociomaterial-Design,* Computer Supported Cooperative Work,
DOI 10.1007/978-3-319-12607-4_3

practices that should be used to determine the correct CTAS score. The ETRIAGE system was designed with the CTAS assessments and guidelines as the fundamental data structure and decision making as in suggesting the urgency level of the patient based upon the type data was also done based upon then CTAS guidelines. While ETRIAGE in principle was intended to support the CTAS processes within the ED, implementing the ETRIAGE in the pediatric ED had a very problematic side effect—namely increasingly large line-ups at the triage station.

When I first arrived in Vancouver, my original research task was to figure out what was wrong with the ETRIAGE system and why it did not work in the pediatric ED. But, before I arrived in Vancouver, the ED manager had taken the decision to retract the ETRIAGE from use, and go back to paper. Understanding the significance of this decision is important, since it was essential in terms of what occurred afterwards. It is quite a brave move for an organization—in this case, a hospital—to realize their error in deciding to buy and implement a digital system, and then to decide that the negative impact of that decision was so large that they had to go back to paper. The decision also changed my post-doctoral research, which then began investigating what was wrong with ETRIAGE after the fact, rather than what was problematic in the practical usage of the system. Many fundamental issues were problematic in the design, but among them was the fundamental understanding of nurses' work when triaging patients, which was embedded in the fundamental design of ETRIAGE (Bjørn and Balka 2007a). ETRIAGE was designed to enforce medical guidelines for triage, but did not take into account that in practice triaging is done with respect for the current status of and the context within the ED. This meant that the decision support and digital algorithms within ETRIAGE did not take into account nurses' expertise on how to triage, causing delays as well as frustrations among nurses (Bjørn and Balka 2007). Experts do not follow guidelines; they simply act and do what is right (Dreyfus 1997). But ETRIAGE enforced guidelines. While analyzing ETRIAGE, I spent many hours in the ED facilities observing the work of nurses, clerks, physicians, housekeeping staff, and all other hospital roles that are critical to make an ED function. In addition, I studied the large number of artefacts and the practices involved with these artefacts such as clipboards, whiteboards, paper templates, etc., which are all part of the coordination of the work in the ED. The ED is open 24 h a day, 7 days a week and is visited by approximately 38,000 patients per year. At all times, there are one to three pediatric physicians with a specialty in emergency medicine present, along with seven to nine registered nurses. Physicians work 8-h shifts, while the nurses work 12-h shifts. In total, there are approximately 75 nurses and 30 medical personnel (from medical students to consultants) employed in the ED. This organizational setup requires much collaboration and coordination—not only within the ED, but also between the ED and other departments in the hospital.

Despite the bad experience with ETRIAGE, the ED was still interested in going digital. In the spring of 2007, the provincial healthcare authority agreed to sponsor a new electronic Emergency Department Information System (EDIS) for the pediatric ED. However, the offer came with restrictions. The ED had to collaborate with the regional health authority, which at the time had a project implementing

EDIS in all regional EDs. This meant that the pediatric ED could not select their own platform; it had to be Cerner FirstNet, which was already implemented in two regional EDs. The pediatric ED had to collaborate with the regional EDs as well as with the regional health authority on the design, since all EDs were supposed to use the same system to ensure the ability to share information across hospitals. The final constraint was that the system had to be implemented by the end of the fiscal year (March 2008), which meant in 10 months time. Working as a researcher in the middle of this large project was a very interesting and challenging task since suddenly my role as the analytical ethnographic researcher was transformed into a participant in a team of nurses and other healthcare professionals, who together were involved in the design and reconfiguration of this new EDIS system. In the period between August 2007 and February 2008, I participated in design workshops organized by the regional health authority together with the Cerner designers and participants from the provincial pediatric ED. My role was not pre-determined (Bjørn and Boulus-Rødje 2011), but something which arose during the process, during which I became very engaged and involved with the design activities by voicing the ED staff's concerns (Bjørn and Boulus-Rødje 2013). The EDIS had two basic components: electronic triage and patient tracking. The electronic triage system was based upon a fundamentally different approach to understanding triage compared to ETRIAGE, in particular the new EDIS system placed the full responsibility of triage decisions on the triage nurse. Also, the collaborative nature of triage work and related aspects such as triage drift were possible to execute in the new system (Bjørn and Rødje 2008). The design of the electronic triage template was an interesting process of negotiation between the different work practices in adult EDs and pediatric EDs. While the initial approach was one of a standardized template for all EDs, the end result through discussions and analysis was recognition of the crucial differences in these medical practices, resulting in the template only being standardized up to a certain point. The template was then divided into two templates and each was customized for the particular context of pediatric triage or adult triage (Bjørn et al. 2009).

The design of the patient tracking component of the EDIS involved a discussion on the current processes as they were handled in the current dry erase whiteboard (Fig. 3.1).

The work thus entailed discussions of the particular processes for inserting an IV or handling the coordination of X-rays with the radiology department, and how the new EDIS could be customized towards supporting these processes, *as well as* how the pediatric ED had to change and accommodate the implementation of the new system in their processes. Since the patient tracking system was to replace the dry erase whiteboards in the ED, the close ethnographic studies of the current use of whiteboards in the ED proved very valuable (Bjørn and Hertzum 2011). During the process, it also became apparent that some current practices, in areas such as housekeeping and nursing breaks, that were organized on the dry erase whiteboard could no longer be handled as part of the whiteboard practices. This is because the digital whiteboard was designed with a patient focus in mind while the existing dry erase whiteboard was designed with a cubicle focus in mind leaving no space for

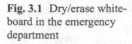

Fig. 3.1 Dry/erase whiteboard in the emergency
department

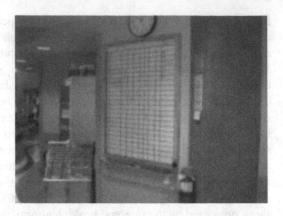

processes such as cleaning. This change in the fundamental focus of the coordinative whiteboard impacted the work processes in the pediatric ED, meaning staff
had to create new processes and additional artefacts (smaller whiteboard and paper
schemes) to accommodate the disconnected practices that were simply remnants
according to the new digital whiteboard. This meant that practices that had been
connected prior to the implementation of the digital whiteboards became disconnected, and thus the healthcare professionals had to take extra steps in combining
the practices across different artefacts.

During the design workshops, I became part of the core group of ED personnel
that referred to itself as the "Fabulous Five," and I was the fifth superhero. My role
as researcher became highly engaged with the concrete problems at hand when
designing a new system. Over the months between July and March, I spent many
hours in design workshops and in the ED looking closely and broadly at practices,
artefacts, and new designs—and, interestingly, I found new ways to provide valuable observations about how the ethnographic accounts that I had created could be
directly relevant to the design of the new EDIS system.

> I found your [the researcher's] role incredibl[y] helpful [...] I find that there were times
> when we got stuck with stuff, that you...framed questions in such a way that they steered us
> to think of things that we were perhaps either stuck with or hadn't considered. And that was
> incredibly helpful because...you are under a lot of pressure to get work done [...]. I think
> the possibility that there would be something published from it—from this department—is
> very [important]... And...expos[ing] people to the opportunity to be involved in some writ-
> ing [...]—that's fantastic. It's the way we should be going, it's the real collaboration—and
> I think the fact that you were seeing it in action versus just interviewing and hearing our
> interpretations of what happened brings a very different light to the whole writing and the
> work. (Emergency department head nurse, November 2008)

After all the design workshops had ended, I was invited to participate in the user
testing, since I was one of only five who actually knew all about the EDIS system and the changed processes. While the new system was a reconfiguration of
a generic EDIS system, we had made very significant changes in the system, as
well as defined many new ways of handling the routine processes within the ED.
Actually, we had made so many changes that the regular staff person from the

vendor company could not conduct the training on the system. However, I declined the offer of the system since I was not a user and was not even trained or educated as a nurse; therefore, I could not accept the responsibility. I was then asked to be part of the training team that was to train the over 100 ED personnel who were to use the EDIS. However, I also declined this offer. Even though I wanted to help, there were challenges in training while preserving the nature of my external role as researcher to observe the results of the system going live. If I were to train users on the system, I would be advocating for the system, which means that I would sacrifice my role as an external researcher that ED staff could openly talk to about their frustrations and difficulties with the system. How could I first train a user on the system, and then later ask the same person to honestly tell me about their experience with the same system?

In March 2008, the new EDIS system went live in the pediatric ED, and it actually went well. I observed the new practices in the first 3 months of use, and then again after 6 months of use, only few unanticipated aspects had emerged—and to my surprise the large number of processes we had defined including both the digital and the physical artefacts actually seemed to work. 4 years later, in August 2012 in Copenhagen, I met one of the members of the "Fabulous Five," a nurse who had been an important part in the design workshops. She still worked in the pediatric ED, and she explained that they still used the system and the processes as we had designed them 4 years ago. Of course, small changes had been made, but the general design and process remained the same. In addition, she also explained to me that they now were in the process on getting digital orders as well as digital X-ray processes—however, I will return to this aspect later in this book.

The design of the EDIS system to support the practices in the Canadian pediatric ED followed the sociomaterial-design approach, as the process involved serious consideration of both the pre-existing and new sociomaterial practices in the ED. However, at the time, I did not explicitly refer to the work as sociomaterial-design. It was not until the years following in reflections upon the work and in my many discussions with fellow researchers—in particular with my co-author Carsten Østerlund during the writing of this book and comparison to our current work—that it became clear to me that the sociomaterial-design approach had been one of the factors for why the large-scale design project of the EDIS in the ED functioned so well and became a success in the eyes of the healthcare professionals who worked with it. We will come back to this topic later and go into more details on what this means in practice.

3.2   The U.S. Emergency Department

Much like the Canadian ED, the American ED nests within a larger pediatric tertiary hospital affiliated with a university. Located in a large U.S. metropolitan area, the ED sees approximately 50,000 children annually ranging from newborns to young adults up to 21 years of age who have pediatric ailments. These children come from all walks of life. Both urban poor and wealthy families seek treatment in the ED. As a Level 1 pediatric trauma center the U.S. ED can handle the most complicated patients and often admits children from other parts of the world.

The ethnographic study of the U.S. ED was part of a larger multi-site investigation of artefacts tracking patients' movements from primary care clinics through to EDs, and inpatient wards to outpatient care. As part of my (Carsten Østerlund) dissertation research I spent the majority of my time from the years 1998 to 2000 in the U.S. ED following doctors, nurses, secretaries, and clerical staff along in their daily work and focused in particular on the practices involved in documenting and tracking patient care (Østerlund 2002; Østerlund 2003; Østerlund 2004; Østerlund 2007; Østerlund 2008a; Østerlund 2008b; Østerlund and Boland 2009).

The purpose of the study was to understand the social and material nature of knowledge sharing within and across healthcare settings. In a previous ethnographic study of an adult ED, I had noticed a great mixture of technologies: some paper-based, others electronic, wall-mounted, or recorded on bed sheets and windows. I wanted to understand how the social and material aspects of these systems were part of the knowledge sharing or lack thereof that occurs between and in the many healthcare settings patients travel to on their way to recovery or, in some cases, over the course of their deteriorating health.

I initially was looking for a place where I could track the implementation of an information system that linked several settings in the hopes of learning if doctors and nurses changed their knowledge sharing practices across settings when encountering the capabilities of new artefacts. My quest to find such a system lead to much frustration and taught me a great deal about the myths and realities of medical information systems, and the social and material bundling of work in healthcare settings.

With help from several medical informatics research centres I started looking for a project that involved the implementation of a system linking healthcare settings across institutional boundaries. I found one initiative that was implementing webcams in neonatal units, allowing parents, and potentially primary care physicians, access to images and information on the patients. As I was about to begin my research, the project was scaled back and became a local project narrowly focused on the neonatal unit with little, if any, external involvement.

My search continued. Repeatedly, I would hear stories about institutions, sometimes in other countries, where great systems were being implemented or had been implemented, but following up on those instances felt very much like chasing a mirage. When I showed up, the system was rarely used and often contained in only one department or clinic. Finally, I conceded that the highly integrative system that the medical informatics community envisioned might not exist, and if it did, I might not be able to find it. With this in mind, I ended up gaining access to the U.S. pediatric ED used in the case study through contacts with physicians developing an early version of what today is known as a personal health record (PHRs). It was a web-based system that allowed parents to send follow-up questions to physicians, check test results, and receive discharge instructions. The designers were interested in feedback on the use of their system in exchange for sponsoring my study.

Once in the ED, I faced a hodgepodge of information systems, in a multitude of sociomaterial stripes and colors. There was no lack of electronic information systems, paper-based forms, tubing systems, filling mechanisms, whiteboards, films, etc. Many of the electronic systems were local, meaning they had been designed by physicians with a knack for computers or purchased to fit a particular group's needs. Given my interest in tracking the artefacts and knowledge sharing associated with patients' movements from primary care clinics through the ED and beyond, I started paying attention to the triage desk where nurses would receive patients—whether they arrived by ambulance or walked off the street. I would follow triage nurses for the 12-h duration of their shift. They started their day flipping through a pile of what they called "expect sheets" that were received from outside caregivers sending patients to the ED. Some were faxed, others were emailed or phoned in. From there, I would follow their work in assessing and sorting the status of all the patients filling up the waiting room or those wheeled directly into a trauma room. In a similar manner, I joined other nurses, doctors, and clerical staff in their daily sociomaterial doings, whether it involved patient care, meetings, administration, or—more typically—a mix of these activities.

My initial sponsors were far from the only ones engaged in design work. I constantly encountered interactions with design: nurses adjusted a triage template, doctors added new fields to an ED note system, changes were made to the discharge note rubrics based on requests from the diabetes clinic, and so forth. Many of these changes affected other sociomaterial practices and led to prolonged negotiations among numerous staffing groups. Rarely did these negotiations involve the hospital's IT staff, who almost quite literally lived their lives on the margin as they were stowed away in a trailer at the edge of the hospital grounds.

About midway through my participant observation in the ED, my sponsors asked me to produce a report on the use of their web-based patient health record linking parents and physicians. Despite months spent in the ED, I had only observed the system used when the designers were around to promote it. Otherwise, it lived a shadow existence on the ED's computer terminals. Doctors reported that the system (along with many other electronic systems) didn't fit into their workflow or their use of other artefacts, and took time away from their patient care. Many noted that they needed more training to effectively use it. Others argued that they disagreed with the type of information shared with patients and the level of detail required by the system. The news was not welcomed. Weeks of dissertation purgatory followed where I had to renegotiate access to the ED and the hospital (Fig. 3.2).

I soon learned that a ward is not a ward to everybody or at all times. What nurses might consider one department under the jurisdiction of one nurse manager, doctors would see as two departments managed by different chief physicians—an illustration of the unique cultures of starkly different sub-disciplines. Often the bundling of practices, artefacts and places changed within a shift, such as when a nurse started out in triage and later moved to fast track. Artefacts played an equally important role in this shifting map. Sometimes an expect sheet marked the actions of the local triage section. At other times, it was a link between primary care doctors and the ED. Depending on what artefact I handled, and whom I talked to and when, different

Fig. 3.2 Ambulance outside
the hospital

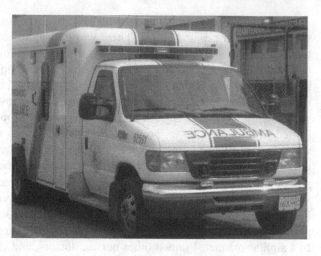

bundles of organizational practices took place. These experiences made me sensitive to the variations among artefacts, doctors, and nurses in terms of how they existed and moved among the divisions in the hospital and beyond.

References

Bjørn, P., Balka, E.: Health care categories have politics too: unpacking the managerial agendas of electronic triage systems. ECSCW 2007. In: Proceedings of the Tenth European Conference on Computer Supported Cooperative Work, Limerick, Ireland, Springer (2007a)

Bjørn, P., Balka, E.: Technology transforms the space for knowledge acquisition. ED-Media, World Conference on Educational Multimedia, Hybermedia and Telecommunication, Vancouver, Canada, ACM (2007b)

Bjørn, P., Boulus-Rødje, N.: Dissenting in reflective conversations: critical components of doing action research. Action Res. J. **9**(3), 282–302 (2011)

Bjørn, P., Boulus-Rødje, N.: Empirical sensibility in design workshops of healthcare infrastructures. In: Ellingsen, G., Bjørn, P. (eds) Infrastructures in Healthcare, Tromsø, University of Tromsø, Norway (2013)

Bjørn, P., Hertzum, M.: Artefactual multiplicity: a study of emergency-department whiteboards. Comput. Support. Coop. Work (CSCW): Int. J. **20**(1), 93 (2011)

Bjørn, P., Rødje, K.: Triage drift: a workplace study in a pediatric emergency department. Comput. Support. Coop. Work (CSCW): Int. J. **17**(4), 395–419 (2008)

Bjørn, P., Burgoyne, S., et al.: Boundary factors and contextual contingencies: configuring electronic templates for health care professionals. Eur. J. Inf. Syst. **18**, 428–441 (2009)

Bullard, M.: CTAS+ or eTriage: taking advantage of the informatics age, slides: The Science of Triage: SAEM, Division of Emergency Medicine, University of Alberta (2003)

Dreyfus, H.: Intuitive, deliberative and calculative models of expert performance. In: Zsambok C., Klein, G. (eds.) Naturalistic Decision Making, pp. 17–28. Lawrence Erlbaum, Mahwah (1997)

Østerlund, C.: Documenting dreams: patient-centered records versus practice-centered records. Sloan School of Management. M.I.T., Cambridge. PhD-thesis (2002)

Østerlund, C.: Documenting practices: the indexical centering of medical records. Outl.: Crit. Soc. Stud. **2**, 43–68 (2003)

Østerlund, C.: Mapping medical work: information practices across multiple medical settings. J.
    Inf. Stud. **3**, 35–44 (2004)
Østerlund, C.: Genre combinations: a window into dynamic communication practices. J. Manage.
    Inf. Syst. **23**(4), 81–108 (2007)
Østerlund, C.: Documents in place: demarcating places for collaboration in healthcare settings.
    Comput. Support. Coop. Work (CSCW): Int. J. **17**(2–3), 7–40 (2008a)
Østerlund, C.: The materiality of communicative practice: the boundaries and objects of an emer-
    gency room genre. Scand. J. Inf. Syst. **20**(1), 7–40 (2008b)
Østerlund, C., Boland, D.: Document cycles: Knowledge flows in heterogenous healthcare infor-
    mation system environments. The 42nd Annual Hawaii International Conference on System
    Science (HICSS-42). Hawaii, HI, IEEE Computer Society Press (2009)

Chapter 4
Analytical Approach to Study Sociomaterial Nature of Artefacts

For the purpose of this book, we wanted to compare the empirical data from our two extensive ethnographic field studies of two pediatric EDs. While in the previous chapter, we presented two narratives of the research engagements with the different field sites, we will now explain in more detail how we methodologically approach the two sites. In addition, and maybe even more importantly, we show how, in the analytical process, we engaged with an enormous amount of rich, in-depth qualitative empirical data from the two sites.

4.1 Ethnography for Design

If we start by exploring how we created and engaged with the empirical data while focusing on the two cases, it becomes clear that our main approach in both cases was ethnography (Orlikowski and Baroudi 1991; Blomberg et al. 1993; Harvey and Myers 1995; Marcus 1995) in the tradition of work place studies and field work for design in particular (Forsythe 1999; Luff et al. 2000; Randall et al. 2007; Suchman 2007), with an interventionist approach (Mesman 2007; Zuiderent-Jerak 2007). But what does that mean?

Ethnography is not a neutral research approach nor is it simply a list of techniques for research. Ethnography is not about how long the researcher spends in the field (Crabtree et al. 2013), nor is just anyone capable of doing ethnography (Forsythe 1999). Ethnography is an approach wherein the researcher engages her or himself as an instrument in the inquiry of exploring a phenomenon. Ethnography is concerned with the everyday and with intimate knowledge from face-to-face interactions with people (Marcus 1995). It requires analytical sensibility as the researcher closely trails people and artefacts in the context of their everyday activities, focusing for instance on the working procedures and practical reasoning of doctors, nurses, patients, and hospital clerical staff and administrators (Bjørn and Boulus-Rødje 2013). In our two empirical studies, we paid particular attention to how participants and technologies, ranging from paper and metal racks to complex

© Springer International Publishing Switzerland 2014
P. Bjørn, C. Østerlund, *Sociomaterial-Design,* Computer Supported Cooperative Work,
DOI 10.1007/978-3-319-12607-4_4

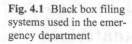

Fig. 4.1 Black box filing systems used in the emergency department

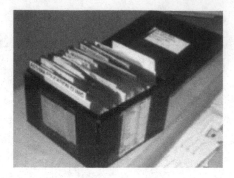

digital information systems, came together in the working procedures and practical reasoning of particular organizational settings (Luff et al. 2000).

Ethnography does not mean that the researcher is passive or a "fly-on-the-wall." Instead, ethnographers get involved with the field over the course of their engagement with it, as did we in the two empirical studies. This means that part of the results of our ethnography were directly visible in the practices that we engaged in—as in the work done in the design workshop focusing on the new EDIS in the Canadian ED. These interventions also became part of the empirical material and observations that were captured in the field notes, in rich descriptions, and in drawings, pictures, recordings, etc (Fig. 4.1). The result of the ethnographic work was manifold and, besides the papers we have published, our ethnographic data took up a lot of space on our hard drives—not to mention the "in-the-head data," which is all the extra knowledge and information about the field that we have acquired during our long-term engagement, but is absent in the descriptions (Randall et al. 2007). When we first met in January 2009, we were curious about the unique possibility of comparing our empirical cases to see where this would lead us. What could we learn about the work practices and use of artefacts within ED work by comparing our efforts that we could not see by simply focusing on the particularities embedded in each case?

4.2   Similarities Across the Empirical Cases

At the most basic levels of comparison—such as time spanned and areas studied—we quickly saw many similarities between the two studies. While each author collected data separately without prior discussions, both studies spanned 2 years of data collection and focused on the emerging practices associated with artefacts and their materiality. The EDs were both pediatric trauma centres associated with teaching hospitals, and each saw approximately 50,000 children a year. Patient tracking systems and their use, development, and implementation played a central role in both studies. The U.S. ED data gathered from 1998 to 2000 were part of a larger multi-site investigation of artefacts tracking patients' movements from primary care clinics through EDs and inpatient wards to outpatient care. The study was particularly relevant as it followed the development and use of patient tracking systems in EDs as they evolved from predominantly paper-based endeavors to whiteboard and early electronic tracking systems. The Canadian study conducted from 2006 to 2008 focused on practices in ED work and how they related to the development and implementation of an electronic triage and patient tracking system. The study was particularly relevant as it engaged with the move from paper- and whiteboard-based patient tracking to the implementation of electronic tracking systems. In both cases, the researcher was granted access to conduct substantial on-site observations and interviews, participate in planning and staff meetings, and analyze archival data.

Historically, few academic publications have integrated ethnographical data from two studies conducted by different researchers. In recent years, however, this approach has been of increasing interest to research on technology, organization, and practices, some of which span radically different organizational contexts (Tyre and Orlikowski 1994; Staudenmayer et al. 2002; Levina and Vaast 2005; Balka et al. 2008). In our case, we conducted studies in EDs of approximately the same size and structure, and focused on the same unit of analysis: doctors,' nurses,' and clerical workers' work practices and use of artefacts. Despite the span in time and location of the two studies, we emerged from the field with similar understandings of the role of artefacts in ED work.

Table 4.1 compares the similarities of the two cases.

Table 4.1 Cross-study comparison

	U.S. pediatric ED	Canadian pediatric ED
Size & type	Tertiary pediatric teaching hospital with Level 1 Pediatric Trauma Centre. Sees ~ 50,000 children/year from birth through 21 years of age	Provincial tertiary pediatric teaching hospital with Level 1 Pediatric Trauma Centre. Sees ~45,000 children/year from birth to 17 years of age
Organizational structure	Two parallel patient tracks: Urgent (17 beds) and fast track (8 beds)	Two parallel patient tracks: acute (17 beds) and fast track (6 beds)
Other sites studied	2 EDs, 5 primary care clinics, 2 inpatient wards	Field trips to 2 other Canadian hospitals
Access to field	Negotiated through a medical informatics research centre at hospital and the hospital's quality improvement office	Part of a large research project, ACTION for Health, with various academic and hospital partners
Field observation	15 months, 4–5 days a week involving more than 2000 h of observation and informal interviews; half in ED	24 months with observations clustered in periods involving approximately 320 h of observation
Semi-structured interviews	45 recorded and 26 transcribed	8 recorded and 8 transcribed
Other data collection methods	5 structured focus group interviews and numerous informal focus group interviews. Numerous meetings, including ED staff meetings, hospital quality improvement group meetings, etc.	22 design workshops of 4–8 h with 3–12 participants, approximately 130 h in total
		One focus group interview
		Phone interview survey with 8 out of 10 pediatric EDs in Canada
		Participation in various hospital meetings

Table 4.1 (continued)

	U.S. pediatric ED	Canadian pediatric ED
Informal contacts	Yes	Yes
Key artefacts	Progress notes, discharge summaries, flow sheets, whiteboards, team and sub-specialty notes, orders, test results, radiology reports, social service forms, referrals to sub-specialties, pharmacy prescriptions, etc.	Yellow notes, triage forms, nurse charts, physician charts, orders, whiteboards, chart racks, clipboards, test results, X-ray orders, etc.
Key technologies	Intranet, Internet, paper, whiteboards, email, telephone, pagers, filing bins and binders, flags, racks, tabletops, magnets	Paper, whiteboards, electronic whiteboards, clipboard, chart racks, laminated paper, magnets, sticky notes, flags, racks, power plugs, tabletops
Unit of analysis	Work practices and use of artefacts among doctors, nurses, and clerks	Work practices and use of artefacts among doctors, nurses, and clerks

4.3   Sociomaterial Analytical Process

Drawing on the relational thinking found in sociomateriality (Schatzki et al. 2001; Law 2004; Østerlund and Carlile 2005; Suchman 2007) and the sensitivity towards artefacts characteristic of work place studies (Luff et al. 2000; Randall et al. 2007), we analyzed and interpreted data from our empirical studies by focusing on how people and artefacts intersected in everyday activities and during critical changes. Inspired by the constant comparison technique found in grounded theory (Glaser and Strauss 1967; Strauss and Corbin 1990), we compared the sociomaterial practices of the artefacts first within each case (longitudinal analysis) and then across the two cases (cross-case analysis).

First, we each digested our ethnographic data by writing small case descriptions following an iterative data interpretation process (Schultze 2000). This resulted in a number of vignettes that constituted our individual interpretation of the data and descriptions of artefacts. These summaries enabled us to become more familiar with each other's data (we were already familiar with our own data) before we attempted to compare across the cases (Eisenhardt 1989).

Second, our conceptualization of artefacts as associated with bounding practices and emerging out of doctors' and nurses' sociomaterial practices formed the basis for comparisons across the cases. Here we identified a complete list of artefacts in each of the EDs, leading to a long list. Based on this mapping, we identified key local coordinative artefacts, defined by artefact critical for making the ED function. This identification was done while in the field by examining the artefact identified to us as the most important, as well as the artefacts we knew from our many observations were critical to make the ED function. In ED work, key artefacts come in many different forms. Key artefacts include the patient chart, the chart racks, the whiteboards, and the clipboards; however, there are also an array of different types of colored documents, such as yellow notes, blue and pink cards, and green sheets. Some of these artefacts become bounded in their association with patients and healthcare professionals, while others are bounded in different ways as they more generically guide the work. Examples of patient-bounded artefacts are patient charts, triage forms, and X-ray forms. The more generically bounded artefacts are, for example, the chart rack or the whiteboard. Each of these artefacts nests within the parts of larger and smaller entanglements. The generically-bound artefacts often form separate boundings embedded within several patient-bounded artefacts. For example, the chart rack connects the various individual patient charts and the whiteboard makes visible the connections between patients' room locations. Some of these artefacts are non-permanent and only exist temporally: They exist with a particular purpose in mind and are then trashed. However, others are permanent records kept during a whole patient stay—or even between admissions. Using the comparative method, we contrasted these artefacts by paying attention to differences across the EDs.

Third, we compared artefacts within cases by (a) looking and their interdependent roles in ED work, particularly patient tracking, and (b) identifying emergent shifts in artefacts and practices within each case. The process allowed us to challenge each other's conclusions and our emergent interpretations.

The more we looked at and compared cases the *less* clearly demarcated became the key artefacts we had initially identified. Where one artefact started and another ended became fuzzy. We started exploring the way we bound practices and artefacts. Practicing this form of "suspicion" (Klein and Myers 1999) embedded in the comparative analysis led us to look for new boundings. What facts of ED work did the doctors and nurses bring to the foreground through their practices and what features did they marginalize? Next, we searched for possible intra-actions among artefacts, artefacts and their locations, and artefacts and people's mobility patterns associated with the different bounding. Finally, we tracked the history of boundings and changes to their intra-actions over time to better understand the dynamic transformations of artefacts in practices and their co-figurations.

The new insights lead us to repeat our three analytical steps: (1) interpretive vignettes, (2) cross-case comparison, and (3) within-case comparison. Not surprisingly, we did find individual coordinative artefacts associated with distinct boundings. It was only the beginning. Doctors and nurses performed many more boundings by shifting the boundaries of what became binded-together and where the [bracketing] practices of what is inside and outside of an artefact over time. We found that healthcare professionals did so by bounding artefacts, locations, and mobility patterns in other ways. Analytically we could describe these bounding in three types: bounding multiple artefacts, bounding artefact and locations, and bounding artefact and people's mobility patterns. Mapping the many boundaries performed helped explain local differences in choices of materiality for particular information systems and how these affected the ongoing debates and conflicts associated with changes to the EDs' patient tracking capabilities.

At this stage in our analytical process, we became certain that we had found a useful conceptualization of how to identify particular critical bounding practices of the phenomenon we study, and how we could offer guidelines on identifying and demonstrating the most relevant boundings related to design of digital artefacts. It is not enough to state the phenomenon as a complex ball of yarn, we need to take into account the design interest and point to which strings to pull out and investigate before taking design decisions for new digital designs. We found that the three boundings that sociomaterial-designers should explore and experiment with when designing digital artefact are the boundings of multiple artefact, locations, and people's movements. In the next chapter, we will dig further and in more detail into each of these boundings to illustrate our point.

References

Balka, E., Bjørn, P., et al.: Steps towards a typology for health informatics. Computer Supported Cooperative Work (CSCW), San Diego, CA, USA, ACM (2008)

Bjørn, P., Boulus-Rødje, N.: Empirical sensibility in design workshops of healthcare infrastructures. In: Ellingsen, G., Bjørn, P. (eds.) Infrastructures in Healthcare. University of Tromsø, Tromsø (2013)

Blomberg, J., Giacomi, J., et al.: Ethnographic field methods and their relation to design. In: Schuler, D., Namioka, A. (eds.) Participatory Design: Principles and Practices, pp. 123–155. Lawrence Erlbaum Associates, London (1993)

Crabtree, A., Tolmie, P., et al.: How many bloody examples do you want? Fieldwork and generalisation. European Conference on Computer Supported Cooperative Work (ECSCW). Springer, Greece (2013)

Eisenhardt, K.M.: Building theories from case study research. Acad. Manage. Rev. 14(4), 532–550 (1989)

Forsythe, D.: It's just a matter of common sense: ethnography as invisible work. Comput. Support. Coop. Work (CSCW): Int. J. 8, 127–145 (1999)

Glaser, B.G., Strauss, A.L.: The Discovery of Grounded Theory; Strategies for Qualitative Research. Aldine, Chicago (1967)

Harvey, L., Myers, M.: Scholarship and practice: the contribution of ethnographic research methods to bridging the gab. Inf. Technol. People 8(3), 13–27 (1995)

Klein, H.K., Myers, M.D.: A set of principles for conducting and evaluating interpretive field studies in information systems. MIS Q. 23(1), 67–92 (1999)

Law, J.: After Method: Mess is Social Science Research. Routledge, London (2004)

Levina, N., Vaast, E.: The emergence of boundary spanning competence in practice: implications for implementation and use of information systems. MIS Q. 29(2), 335–363 (2005)

Luff, P., Hindmarch, J., et al. (eds.): Workplace Studies: Recovering Work Practice and Informing System Design. Cambridge University Press, Cambridge (2000)

Marcus, G.: Ethnography in/of the world system: the emergence of multi-sited ethnography. Annu. Rev. Anthropol. 24, 95–117 (1995)

Mesman, J.: Disturbing observations as a basis for collaborative research. Sci. Cult. 16(3), 281–295 (2007)

Orlikowski, W.J., Baroudi, J.: Studying information technology in organizations: research approaches and assumptions. Inf. Syst. Res. 2(1), 1–28 (1991)

Østerlund, C., Carlile, P.: Relations in practice: sorting through practice theories on knowledge sharing in complex organizations. Inf. Soc. 21(2), 91–107 (2005)

Randall, D., Harper, R., et al.: Fieldwork for Design: Theory and Practice. Springer, London (2007)

Schatzki, T.R., Knorr-Cetina, K., et al. (eds.): The Practice Turn in Contemporary Theory. Routledge, London (2001)

Schultze, U.: A confessional account of an ethnography about knowledge work. MIS Q. **24**(1), 3–6 (2000)

Staudenmayer, N., Tyre, M., et al.: Time to change: temporal shifts as enablers of organizational change. Organ. Sci. **13**(5), 583–597 (2002)

Strauss, A., Corbin, J.M.: Basic of Qualitative Research: Grounded Theory Procedures and Techniques. Sage, London (1990)

Suchman, L.A.: Human–Machine Reconfigurations: Plans and Situated Actions. Cambridge University Press, Cambridge (2007)

Tyre, M.J., Orlikowski, W.J.: Windows of opportunity: temporal patterns of technological adaptation in organizations. Organ. Sci. **5**(1), 98–118 (1994)

Zuiderent-Jerak, T.: Preventing implementation: exploring interventions with standardization in healthcare. Sci. Cult. **16**(3), 311–329 (2007)

Chapter 5
Bounding Practices

In this chapter, we present the results of our analytical process, untangling the dynamic boundaries for the key artefacts that organize the work in the Canadian and U.S. EDs. The process strives to illuminate the sociomaterial nature of the artefacts by affirming that those artefacts are always part of larger and smaller entanglements. Each of these entanglements constitutes a sociomaterial artefact in its own right—part of the bounding practices providing a distinct order to the ED world and allowing doctors and nurses to perform different sociomaterial practices. In short, the artefacts we untangle are not pre-given but bound up in multiple orderings. We think about the unpacking of sociomaterial practices related to key artefacts as a three-step process, during which we slowly open up to show the complexity that working within a relations epistemology provides. However, instead of simply diving deep into all the complexities of each artefact, we have decided to slowly unpack the bounding practices in the EDs over the next three chapters. This serves the purpose of providing a point of introduction for Ada and Alan in terms of a discussion of how to think relationally when designing artefacts, and what it means to design artefacts without clear boundaries. Alan might feel that the three steps reduce the sociomaterial complexity of artefacts by bracketing out important sociomaterial practices while only attending to the bounding of, for example, multiple artefacts. We ask that Alan stay on track and follow us along to the end when we open up and bring together the different forms of boundings to see how we then bring back together the multiple boundings.

We first start out by examining how practitioners routinely bound multiple artefacts into new artefacts constituting their own boundings, their own ordering of the ED. Second, we investigate the way doctors and nurses bound artefacts and location, again performing distinct bounding practices. Third, we explore how practitioners bound artefacts and their own movements into sociomaterial orders.

Avoiding the illusion that artefacts are pre-given becomes especially pertinent when engaging in sociomaterial-design. The transformation from, for example, a paper-based artefact to a digital artefact can cause a ripple through the entire sociomaterial entanglement, however we will turn to that in a later chapter.

© Springer International Publishing Switzerland 2014   65
P. Bjørn, C. Østerlund, *Sociomaterial-Design,* Computer Supported Cooperative Work,
DOI 10.1007/978-3-319-12607-4_5

5.1   Bounding Multiple Artefacts

Medical documents in the U.S. and Canadian emergency rooms rarely stand alone. One finds piles of documents organized in binders, racks, and bins from the triage desk at the front entrance, through registration, to the patient and chart rooms. Doctors and nurses constantly compile, separate, compare, and shuffle those documents. As they do so, the purpose of those documents, piles, and practices change, as do doctors' and nurses' expectations of content and formatting features. For instance, the triage desk in the U.S. ED utilizes a letter-sized paper form known as the "expect sheet." When an outside entity, for example, a general practitioner is sending a patient to the ED they can fax, email, or call in "an expect sheet." In these documents, a primary care doctor, another hospital, an ambulance, or a helicopter service will record the patient's personal identifiers and a brief history, followed by a list of things they would like to happen to the patient. Those non-ED caregivers are intending to communicate their actions and intentions regarding the particular patient. In the ED, however, the triage nurse places the incoming expect sheets in a bin next to the phone and fax machines. Very little organized effort is put into transferring them to the patient's chart. By the time expect sheets are transferred to the patient's chart, the nurse and physicians are typically well along in their care. Instead, expect sheets are initially enacted as a *pile* rather than as a number of single documents. The practitioners no longer engage with the single piece of paper, but with the "set of papers"—they become *one* artefact: the [expect-sheet-pile]. The bounding, as in binding-together while bracketing out, of the artefact as a pile rather than one piece of paper is critical for ED work. Attending doctors and charge nurses facilitating the overall flow of patients through the U.S. ED regularly frequent the [expect-sheet-pile] by glancing at the bin to determine the size of the pile. The size of the pile in the bin provides the ED practitioners with important information about expected patients. The pile as a coordinative artefact informs the ED personnel about the future status of the ED: Will they be swamped with patients in the next couple of hours, or will it be quieter? Based on their interpretation of the [expect-sheet-pile], the ED personnel will then act accordingly. Staff members simply assess the size of the pile. A tall pile indicates a busy day ahead. A short stack suggests a more leisurely pace. As an example, returning from a round of the in-boxes, one triage nurse is asked by his colleague: "How does it look?" As an answer, the triage nurse holds up his hand, making a four-inch space between his thumb and index finger. The other nurse shakes her head in resignation. In this way, it is not the single expect sheet that constitutes the coordinative artefact; it is the [expect-sheet-pile] that forms the coordinative artefact. In short, the artefact does not have pre-given boundaries as in one sheet of paper but always is part of larger and smaller entanglements—in this case the bounding of multiple artefacts making the pile (Fig. 5.1).

Investigating the Canadian ED, we found a similar dynamic in the triage area, in this instance, facilitating the management of patients waiting to be triaged. Each time a patient enters the front door the triage nurse interrupts her current activity and takes a yellow note from her desk. She time stamps the yellow note in

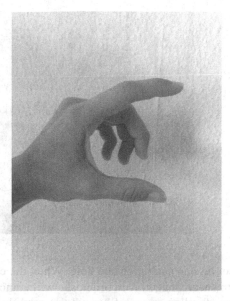

Fig. 5.1 Reconstruction of triage nurse hand indicating busyness in form of the size of the [expect-sheet-pile] artefact

a time-stamping machine on her tabletop, turns to the patient, and asks, "Are you here for emergency, and what seems to be the problem?" The patient and/or the accompanying adult will present the chief complaint, and, based on the busyness in the ED at the current time and the urgency of the chief complaint, the patient will either be called in for a triage interview right away or be asked to wait in the waiting area. If the patient is asked to wait, the triage nurse will place the yellow note on her tabletop and continue with the work of assessing patients, which was interrupted by the arrival of this new patient. During busy times, the triage nurse will have a long queue of yellow notes on her tabletop, each representing a patient waiting to be triaged. The queue will be organized according to the time of arrival (based on the time stamp) and the urgency of the chief complaint (written on the yellow note). In some situations the triage nurse will re-organize the queue of yellow notes based on the chief complaints to make sure the urgently ill patients are seen first. If other triage nurses arrive at the triage area to help out, they will start to call up patients for triage interviews based on the queue of yellow notes on the tabletop (Fig. 5.2).

The bounding associated with the yellow notes takes different forms. First, the yellow note as one piece of paper represents a patient waiting to be triaged, and the information written on the yellow note helps the triage nurse make sense of the urgency and chief complaint of the particular patient. Second, the yellow note is part of a larger artefact that includes the nurses' engagement with the all the yellow notes on the table. The [queue-of-yellow-notes] becomes one entity and serves as one coordinative artefact. The triage nurses act on the queue, a group of

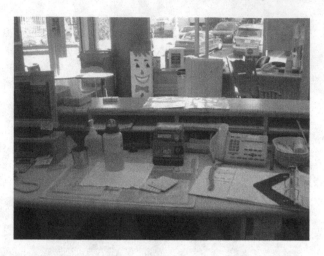

notes and patients, not on one patient or one note. When the charge nurse makes
her round in the ED to ensure that all is in order, she will glance at the triage desk
and assess the [queue-of-yellow-notes]. She will not read the individual yellow
notes but rather will perform the yellow notes as one assemblage, one artefact. If
the queue is long, resources will be re-organized within the ED and more hands
will be assigned to the triage area. The status of the ED can change dramati-
cally at any time, from a few non-urgent patients to an overwhelming number of
gravely ill children. A full waiting room does not necessarily mean that the triage
nurses are overworked and need help. The patients may already have been triaged.
Thus, the bottleneck might be in terms of bedside nurses or examination rooms.
A [long-queue-of-yellow-notes], however, is a clear indication of a triage bottleneck. Without interrupting a busy triage nurse, the charge nurse simply glances
at the carefully organized queue. Many yellow notes mean more resources; few
notes mean the resources are adequate.

As in the case of the expect sheet, the yellow notes can be performed individu-
ally or as a set of yellow notes, and it is only by investigating the boundings created
by the practitioners that we can identify what artefact is at play, and thus whether we
as sociomaterial-designers should think about the artefact as one [piece-of-paper],
or as a "pile" or "queue"? (Fig. 5.3).

To avoid approaching artefacts as pre-given, the sociomaterial-designer must as
a first step investigate how practitioners *bound multiple artefacts*. How are different
sets of artefacts performed as one entity? These "larger" artefacts do not have to assemble objects of the same type, which was the case in the [expect-sheet-pile] and
the [queue-of-yellow-notes]. The elements can be of different types: for example,
a [whiteboard-and-a-chart-rack] bound together, which assist in tracking patients.
The key idea is to approach artefacts as related to other artefacts and explore which
new meanings emerge through the new relations.

Fig. 5.3 Pile of *yellow* notes

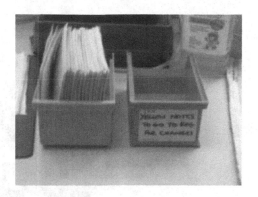

5.2 Bounding Artefact and Locations

Coordinative artefacts in EDs engage in dynamic intra-actions not only with other artefacts but also with their location. Artefacts like paper-based nursing charts or triage templates are mobile and can be placed in different locations within the ED. The location of such artefacts adds a new dimension to how healthcare practitioners perform sociomaterial structures. Locations become important elements of doctors' and nurses' boundings where the entity might be the [artefact-within-the-location]. If we as sociomaterial-designers hope to understand how practitioners assemble artefacts, we must investigate the ways in which they *bound artefacts and locations*. Depending on where an artefact is located within the ED, it becomes a different artefact, part of a new order associated with other practices. We will provide two examples of this phenomenon from the two studies.

In the U.S. ED, the flow sheet constitutes one key artefact. The flow sheet has a purpose similar to the yellow note in the Canadian ED, as both are initiated upon patient arrival. However, whereas the yellow note is trashed after the patient is registered by the registration clerk, the flow sheet stays in the ED as long as the patient. The flow sheets are initiated by triage nurses and change location four times. Each location engages a different set of participants at different times in the patient's care trajectory, combines the location with different documents, and highlights different content. The intra-actions between the artefact and its physical location take on great importance.

First, a triage nurse initiates a flow sheet for every new patient entering the ED. The triage nurse places the new flow sheet in a rack outside the triage examination room, where it is clearly visible from the triage desk but not from the waiting room. The triage nurses sort the flow sheets so that they serve as a sorted list for the order in which to call up patients for their initial physical exam. In this enactment the [flow-sheet-in-a-rack-at-triage] constitutes the artefact (Fig. 5.4).

Second, the flow sheet moves to a gray rack in the main ED, where it is clearly visible from the charting area at the centre of the ED close to the large whiteboard. In the gray rack, the staff arranges the flow sheets according to the patients' perceived urgency and in what part of the ED they should be seen. This adds up to a map of

Fig. 5.4 Chart rack with
clipboards

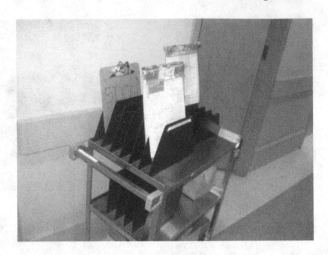

the patients in the waiting room and an itinerary for future activities—who to call
in next. At this time, the artefact becomes [flow-sheet-in-a-gray-rack-in-main-ED].

Third, the flow sheet is placed together with a host of other documents in a box
outside the room assigned to the patient. At this point, the flow sheet's physical location brings it into a field of action dominated by the doctors and nurses caring for
this particular patient. The artefact's proximity to the patients and their significant
others make them potential participants in its use. It is not uncommon to see parents
of a sick child flip through the flow sheet and other documents compiled in the box.
The artefact becomes [flow-sheet-in-a-box].

Fourth, the flow sheet follows the patient, if admitted, or it ends up at the registration desk in a pile of discharged patients, where a registration clerk uses them
when contacting primary care doctors to obtain authorization for insurance purposes. Here we see that depending on the patient trajectory the artefact either becomes
[flow-sheet-of-admitted-patient] or [flow-sheet-at-registration]. In each of these
situations, doctors and nurses perform different boundings, each configuring the
sociomaterial practices of the ED. Finally, the flow sheet will end up in the patient's
medical record, hidden away in the bowels of the hospital and only accessible to
authorized personnel, with the final cut being [flow-sheet-in-medical-record].

In each location, the flow sheet becomes part of a larger coordinative artefact
stipulating the field of action for the relevant participants at that particular mo-
ment in time. The artefact becomes part of different groups' fields of action and
provides a different temporal and spatial reference point for staff members, whether
for newly arrived patients, the waiting room, the patients currently under care, or
patients now gone. Because of the way staff members time their intra-actions with
the artefact while approaching the content of the artefact (as in reading, writing,
etc.), the sociomaterial matter of the artefact not only comprises the bounding of
multiple artefacts, but includes locations such as [flow-sheet-on-clipboard], [flow-
sheet-on-clipboard-in-chart-rack], etc. The sociomateriality practices are continuously changing and bring different meaning to the field of action. Locations are

essential elements in the bounding performed by doctors and nurses. What appears as one artefact at first glance, in fact, constitutes multiple artefacts depending on the location. As sociomaterial-designers, we must stretch our analytical muscles and re-gard locations as important elements of an artefact. Here, the physical layout of the space matters, as does the physicality of the flow sheet. But the physical layout and the physicality of the sheet cannot be seen apart from doctors' and nurses' practices bringing these boundings to life.

In the Canadian ED, there were also several artefacts resembling the flow sheet; however, to show a very different kind of artefact, the [green-X-ray-sheet] from the Canadian case. In the Canadian ED, a coordinative artefact known as the [green-X-ray-sheet] has been designed to assist nurses in finding patients in the waiting room who have recently returned to the ED from the radiology department. The [green-X-ray-sheet] is a laminated, reusable letter-sized piece of paper with a plastic envelope attached in the upper left corner. The sheet is pre-printed with "Emergency Depart-ment, Radiology Exam Completed" in five different languages (Fig. 5.5).

Patients arriving with a chief complaint that requires X-ray examination, such as a fractured wrist (typically a fast-track patient), will be called into a fast-track examination room in the ED after triage, where the physician will decide whether to order an X-ray. The physician or the nurse will then telephone the radiology de-partment to let them know that they have a patient waiting. Meanwhile, the patient is asked to go to the ED waiting room so that other patients can be examined in the fast-track examination room. The patient is dispatched to the radiology department where X-rays are performed, and then goes back to the ED waiting room. Before sending the patient back, a staff person at the radiology department will hand the pa-tient the [green-X-ray-sheet] and radiology staff will place the patient information, such as name and hospital number, in the plastic envelope. This means that at the

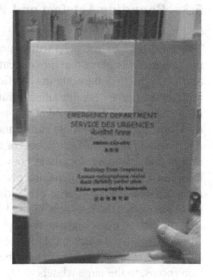

Fig. 5.5 *Green* laminated x-ray sheet

radiology department the [green-X-ray-sheet-at-the-radiology-department] means that an ED patient has been X-rayed and can return to the ED. If the patient is, for example, a clinic patient, then the patient will not get a green-X-ray-sheet, since this is *only* for ED patients. Returning to the ED waiting room, the ED patient will be carrying the [green-X-ray-sheet]. A new sociomaterial artefact therefore emerges: [patient-with-green-X-ray-sheet-in-ED-waiting-room].

Bounding artefact and locations makes it easy for nurses to locate returning X-ray patients simply by scanning the waiting area for signs of green. Obviously, the nurses could have called out the patients' names, but the prevalence of non-English- or French-speaking patients makes this strategy undesirable (as illustrated by the five languages on the green sheet). Instead, the ED staff searches for the green laminated plastic envelopes serving as beacons in a sea of waiting patients. The performances associated with the artefact cannot be fully comprehended in isolation; they come to life only when seen in dynamic intra-actions with the locations in which they are used. The intra-actions between the [green-X-ray-sheet] and the patient holding it cannot be separated when investigating sociomaterial practices. Only by bounding [patient-with-green-X-ray-sheet-in-ED-waiting-room] can we understand doctors' and nurses' bounding practices—namely, that this patient needs to be called into a fast-track examination room for further examination. The clear connection between the green sheet and the patient who returned from radiology would not have been visible to the nurses if the completed X-ray results were simply a flag on a computer screen, since the sociomateriality of the computerized "return from radiology" would be disconnected from the locations. As sociomaterial-designers we must ask how the practitioners create particular boundings of artefact and locations, providing essential information about the sociomaterial performances we hope to support.

5.3   Bounding Artefact and People's Movements

The third type of entanglement bounds artefacts with people's movements. It is not the artefacts alone that move locations; ED personnel move, too. Coordinative artefacts tend to congregate in specific areas. In both EDs one finds document-rich areas at the triage desk, the administration desk, and in the charting area at the heart of the ED, where doctors and nurses tend to access and write their notes on laptops, desktops, paper forms, note cards, and whiteboards. In many situations, however, doctors and nurses move to access or combine documents. For instance, the charge nurses and attending doctors in both the U.S. and Canadian EDs constantly move between different piles of documents. As described above, they will go to the triage area and look at the [queue-of-yellow-notes] (Canada) or [pile-of-expect-sheets] (U.S.) to assess the busyness of the ED. However, this is but one stop. In the U.S. ED, the charge nurse and attending physicians do not do rounds simply by moving from patient to patient, but they move from the triage area documents to stops at the flow-sheet rack in the main ED and bins containing patient charts outside examination rooms, to the large whiteboard in the centre of the ED.

By combining each of these piles of documents, they develop a sense of the overall flow of patients through the ED: How many patients are currently in the waiting room? How far along in the examination and treatment process are patients in the individual exam rooms? What exam rooms can be freed up quickly? How many patients are in need of urgent attention? What doctors and nurses need help? What we see here is that the sociomaterial practices enacting the artefacts (the various piles of documents in various locations) are not only bounded with their locations, they are also bounded with the way the piles of documents become visible for the ED physicians as they *move* through their rounds. The first entity could be [physician-at-triage-desk-accessing-pile-of-expect-sheets], the second entity could be [physician-accessing-flow-sheet-rack-in-main-ED], and the third entity could be [physician-accessing-whiteboard-at-centre-of-ED]. By following the doctors' and nurses' movements, we see how artefacts and locations are part of larger actions which in and of themselves constitute sociomaterial practices that perform particular boundings bringing order to the mangle (Fig. 5.6).

We find a similar example in the acute area of the Canadian case, where the patient chart is divided into two clipboards to accommodate the different mobility patterns of nurses versus physicians. When a patient is assigned to the acute track of the ED, the collective patient chart arrives in a bin at the nursing station where the charge nurse will pick it up and divide the content onto two clipboards. The first clipboard is what the charge nurse will bring with her when calling up the patient and following the patient to the acute examination room. This clipboard contains the nursing notes, and the charge nurse places the clipboard on the wall in the patient examination room. At the acute site in the Canadian ED, patients stay in the same room during their stay and, as such, the clipboard with the nursing notes stays

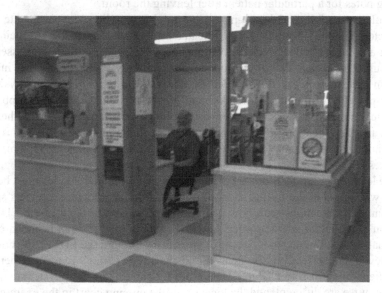

Fig. 5.6 Triage nurse at the triage desk

in the patient room with the patient. (The opposite is true of the fast track, where patients are sent back and forth between various examination rooms and the waiting room, as described in the case of X-ray.) The clipboard with physicians' notes is placed by the charge nurse in the chart rack labeled "Not Seen by Physician" found in the physician area. When ready to see a new patient, a physician will select the first in the queue of patients, indicated by the order of the chart rack, and then move to the whiteboard at the nursing station just next to the physician area to identify the patient's room number before going to find the patient. After completing the exam and filling out the chart and orders, the physician goes to the charge nurse desk to drop off the clipboard in another chart rack labeled "Orders." The physician might then stop for a chat with the nurses about the patient's condition or move back to the physicians' charting area to select a new patient from the chart rack. Handling medical orders by the nurses and ED clerical staff involves even more *patterns of movement*, bringing the staff in proximity to various document systems.

The mobility patterns of doctors and nurses play a central role in their boundings. Artefacts and locations form actionable entities but they often have to be seen in relation to the participants' mobility patterns. In the nurses' case, the [clipboard-with-nursing-notes-and-the-patient-room] bound artefact and location. However, the [clipboard-with-nursing-notes] is also bound to the nurses' mobility patterns, as the nurses constantly walk in and out of the patient rooms while making notes about the status of the patient in the nursing note. The nurses' movements in and out of the patient rooms holding the clipboard with their notes constitute the sociomaterial practices enacting the artefact and perform dynamic boundings of the artefact. The setup allows nurses to constantly check the status of several patients located in different rooms without carrying all the nursing notes at all times, or needing to remember to bring the right clipboard into the right room or what to write in the nursing notes for a particular patient after leaving the room.

Similarly, the [clipboard-with-physician-note] cannot be seen as separate from the doctors' mobility patterns. The physicians on duty are responsible for seeing the patient and taking action, and then waiting until the action is done and assessing the result. This means that physicians do not randomly visit patients, but instead perform a stepwise work flow guided by the way the [clipboard-with-physician-note-is-placed-in-different-chart-racks] and by the particular order the clipboards are sorted in the chart racks. This stepwise mobility pattern intra-acts with the clipboards and their locations. If we as designers start changing these entities, it ripples through the entire sociomaterial entity and changes the conditions for sociomaterial practices.

The location of artefacts not only specifies which particular actions must be taken (as we argued in the former section), the location of particular artefacts stands in dynamic intra-actions with how people logically move around in the ED. The location of particular artefacts often guides the mobility patterns of healthcare professionals. Predicting the movements of physicians through the ED and the hospital is achieved most effectively by focusing on the artefacts they frequent rather than the patients they rush to examine. The mobility patterns of the physician and the bedside nurse are different, and the location of the nursing chart in the examination room and the physician chart in the physician area support these different intra-actions. The sociomateriality of the physician chart is engaged in two highly inter-linked intra-actions—one as the chart moves between the chart racks indicating new patients or new orders, and another as the physician moves between the chart racks, the whiteboards, and the patient examination rooms. Both of these relationships are part of the boundings, and both must be taken into consideration if we are to design new information systems where the artefacts (e.g., the physician chart) go digital.

When we as sociomaterial-designers investigate a nexus of practices, we must try to pluck at the strings of the entanglement and play a little cat's cradle if we hope to avoid approaching artefacts as pre-given but always part of larger and smaller entanglements. Practitioners create different dynamic boundings in their world. While we acknowledge that practitioners can perform an infinite number of boundings, we argue that mapping the intra-actions among named artefacts, locations, and mobility patterns allows us to identify essential sociomaterial performances relevant for the design of artefacts. A three-step analytical process helped us track important cuts in the entanglement by investigating intra-actions among (1) multiple artefacts, (2) artefacts and locations, and (3) artefacts and people's movements.

We have now explored the existing practices of artefacts within ED practices, before even thinking about new design interventions. However, what then happens when we start to think about replacing and changing the pre-existing artefact with new future digital design?

In our next chapter, we will turn to how the sociomaterial practices are impacted by new designs by using as an example the Canadian ED where the paper-based triage form was transformed into a digital triage form.

Chapter 6
Transforming the Sociomateriality of the Triage Template: Canadian ED

In the Canadian ED, one essential artefact is the triage template. The triage template is used during the triage interview during which the triage nurse assesses the urgency of the patient's condition while documenting indicators such as airway, breathing, circulation, weight, temperature, etc. As part of the larger EDIS project, the paper-based triage template was replaced with a digital triage template. The paper-based triage template came in three different versions: one for psychiatric patients, one for acute patients, and one for fast-track patients. Each version has a number of fields to be filled out and *on the back* of the triage template the fields for documenting the nursing notes are pre-printed. In practice, this means that the paper-based triage template is used on the one side to document the triage assessment and on the other side to document the nursing intervention throughout the patient's stay in the ED.

The paper-based triage template intra-acts with the nursing note on the other side of the sheet and constitutes the bounding of the two in one artefact. Being pre-printed on the same piece of paper is essential for the existing design. We have two distinct artefacts (triage template and nursing note), but also one distinct artefact: [triage-template-and-nursing-note]. The details recorded at triage followed the patient all through his or her stay in the ED since the nurses can, at any time, simply turn the paper over and find information such as weight, reason for stay, or vital signs recorded at the time of entry at the ED. The entanglements do not stop with the intra-actions between the nursing note and the triage template. By attaching the [triage-template-and-nursing-note] to a clipboard, the nurses potentially bound a host of other documents allowing for other intra-actions and, thus, boundings.

The clipboard, and with it the triage form and nursing note, travels through the ED. Location and mobility matter for these sociomaterial practices and become an integrative part of the artefacts emerging out of the entanglement. The clipboards are placed within changing chart racks, each intra-acting with their particular location. At the fast-track site of the Canadian ED, one chart rack holds clipboards of patients who have finished particular examination tests such as X-rays or blood tests. Other chart racks hold clipboards of patients whose orders have yet to be done, for example, if nurses have to collect urine samples. And other racks hold clipboards

© Springer International Publishing Switzerland 2014
P. Bjørn, C. Østerlund, *Sociomaterial-Design,* Computer Supported Cooperative Work,
DOI 10.1007/978-3-319-12607-4_6

of patients waiting to be placed in particular rooms, such as the suture room. What healthcare practitioners bound, between what they have to do, and when and where cannot be seen apart from the sociomaterial practices that include the artefacts' assembled, for example, out of the clipboard (including the triage form) and its changing locations. By bounding artefacts and locations, nurses perform different boundings supporting different enactments of the world.

The sociomaterial practices associated with the paper-based triage template cannot be understood from a design perspective without taking into account the way doctors and nurses bound artefacts and people's movements. During busy periods when there is a queue of patients waiting to be registered by the clerk, the triage nurse, will leave the triage desk after finishing the triage interview and walk over to the registration clerk, personally handing the triage template to the registration clerk. This ensures that, even though multiple patients are lining up for registration, the order of the patients based on their time of arrival and urgency is kept up-to-date at all times. On the table of the registration clerk, the order of patients as decided by the triage nurse is documented according to the order of filled out triage interview templates. In cases when the arriving patient enters the ED on a stretcher along with paramedics, the triage nurse simply reaches for the paper-based triage template and walks toward the stretcher to document the assessment in the middle of the triage area, rather than on the blue bench at the triage desk. In this way, the boundings associated with the paper-based triage template enables various intra-actions to occur seamlessly in the practices of the ED personnel.

Designing and implementing an electronic triage template causes ripples through existing boundings. This happened in the Canadian case, where the triage template was made digital while preserving the rest of the sociomaterial setup. This change had consequences. First, the new design disassembled the [triage-template-and-nursing-note] artefact by making the triage template digital while keeping the nursing notes on paper. Also, the digital triage template disconnected the intra-action between the triage template and the clipboard, since it was no longer possible to place the triage template on the clipboard. The clipboard was no longer the artefact it used to be. If ED staff hoped to perform the old boundings associated with the clipboard, they would have to perform extra activities to "connect" the digital triage template and the clipboard, for example, by bringing the clipboard to a computer, looking up the triage template, and comparing it with the other papers; the connection could no longer be made simply by browsing documents on the clipboard. By being unable to place the digital triage template on the clipboard, the opportunity to bound the template with locations was also lost since the digital artefact was always "located" within the computer. This meant it was not possible to move it around in chart-racks, to grab it and triage a patient in a stretcher, or to walk to the registration clerk to make sure the order of patient was kept. We should mention that the digital triage template was available from several computers around the ED, and that COWS (cardex-on-wheels) were also implemented to accommodate mobility, however, less successfully.

The new design of the EDIS system made it possible for the clerks to access the list of patients whose triage interviews were completed, as well as to access the digital triage template on their screens. The order of the patients waiting for registration was also displayed for the clerk, ensuring the problem of keeping the correct order of patients would be solved by the new IT system. However, one problem disrupted this process. The order of patients displayed at registration was sorted by the time the triage interview was initiated. This time stamp was automatically calculated by the system when the triage nurse opened the digital triage template. However, in the ED, they had always kept track of the time of arrival for each patient. This was done by the triage nurse time stamping the yellow note as soon as she noticed a patient entering the ED. As we know from the queue of yellow notes, at busy times the triage interview and the time of arrival are not the same time. The time of arrival is the time stamp on the yellow note, but if the triage nurse is busy and cannot conduct the triage interview right away, she will simply put the yellow note on the table, creating a queue of waiting patients. Now, the ED wanted to have access to the time of arrival at the triage template (as prior to the digital triage template), and that meant that the nurse would override the "time-of-triage-interview" number with the "time-stamp-from-the-yellow-note." The consequence of this action was that the sorted order at registration was no longer the order by which the triage nurse finished the triage interviews and sent them to registration—instead the order was re-sorted based on the time the patient arrived in the ED. Thus, in the cases where a patient needing more urgent care arrived and was pushed forward in the queue of waiting patients, the order by which the clerk would call the patient would still be based on arrival time. This was unacceptable (Fig. 6.1).

The disconnections created by the digital triage template were problematic. To accommodate this decoupling, the ED personnel began printing out the electronic triage template at a printer next to registration as soon as it was typed. This workaround made it possible for the nurses to re-establish the [triage-template-and-nursing-note] artefact by feeding the printer with paper with pre-printed nursing notes on the backside. Moreover, it also made it possible to re-assemble the electronic template and the clipboard, since the printout easily could be attached to the clipboard. Finally, the ED personnel also found that by printing the digital triage templates as soon as they had finished the triage interview, the order of papers in the printer would be the right order for the registration clerk. Since the printer was

Fig. 6.1 Printer at the registration desk

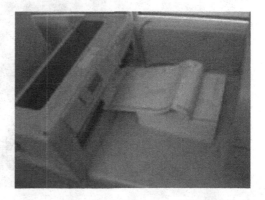

next to the registration clerk, the clerk simply reached out and followed the queue in the printer rather than the one on the screen—and as such the order in the printer overruled the order created by the system. In this way, the sociomaterial practices of bounding artefacts, artefacts and locations, and artefacts and people's movements was reconfigured.

The workaround concerning printing re-established several boundings essential for making the ED function; however, it also created problems. Above we focused on larger entanglements. If we instead investigate the sociomaterial practices associated with a smaller entanglement—the digital triage template—we see that the bounding associated with the digital artefact became interrupted. The electronic triage template was not designed for printing, so the essential order of information fields on the template, which was carefully designed to clearly specify a particular order of vital signs assessment during triage interviews, was disrupted and printed in a coincidental order. The careful design of the electronic template to guide the nurses in assessing airway, breathing, and circulation first and in that order, as well as to make the results of the triage assessment score immediately visible with a simple glance at the computer screen (because the assessment score was recorded on the top of the screen in a large, visible square) totally disappeared in the printed version.

The printed version resembled a matrix printout where the information was printed from the top left corner and down as a long, vertical list, all in the same typeface on letter-sized paper. The order of the information was displaced in terms of typed information, which was problematic. For example, the assessment score was the last information to be entered into the electronic triage template, so it appeared at the bottom of the printout. This meant that in cases where a considerable amount of information was recorded, the assessment score might be printed on page 3. So, to accommodate the bounding associated with multiple artefacts, artefact and locations, and artefact and people's movements, the "printout workaround" was introduced. While this did accommodate certain issues and did re-connect important

Fig. 6.2 Location of the digital whiteboard at the nurses station

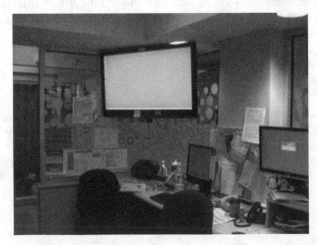

sociomaterial practices, it also disrupted the enacting of the triage template information. This situation could have been addressed at the design stage if the sociomaterial practices surrounding the triage template had been noticed early on and taken into account (Fig. 6.2).

In short, going from paper-based to digital transforms the sociomaterial entanglement and the work it takes to perform productive artefacts. By paying attention to the sociomaterial practices created by the participants when bounding artefacts, locations, and people's movements, we can map the larger and smaller entanglements that are highly relevant for successful sociomaterial-design.

Chapter 7
Negotiating Boundings: New Order Flags in U.S. ED

The dynamic bounding of artefacts, locations, and people's mobility doesn't merely surface when introducing large systems such as the EDIS in the Canadian ED. As a coordinative artefact changes or a new artefact gets introduced, the alteration inevitably leads to deliberations and often conflicts about what intra-actions best support particular agential cuts. Such negotiations monopolize most departmental staff meetings, whether in the ED, inpatient wards, or the primary care clinics. At first glance, such meetings appear to be an unorganized as workplace meetings. This is in fact, is how many ED staff members feel about the meetings and is why they do not bother to show up. Nevertheless, the jagged course of such debates points to the importance staff members ascribe to the bounding practices they perform on a daily basis. To ensure coordination among doctors, nurses, and secretaries, these groups continuously tweak their work along with the bounding of artefacts, locations, and people's movements. These changes lead to conflicts, as they bring to light the stark contrasts between the very performances that constitute doctors' and nurses' work and the power positions in the ED.

The introduction of a new order flag in the U.S. ED illustrates such sociomaterial deliberations. During a routine ED staff meeting, five nurses, two secretaries, and two physicians discuss, among other things, how to best call attention to new orders to improve coordination among doctors and nurses. In the ED library, the nursing manager, Joyce, starts the ED staff meeting. As an experiment, the department recently installed red and green plastic flags mounted on the doorframe of team A's patient rooms (one team among three in the acute area of the ED). The doctors promoted the initiative. Usually, when doctors write orders to nurses, they place their orders in the bins found outside each patient room. On team A, the doctors are now supposed to flip out a red or green flag and thereby signal to the nurses that they have an urgent or "emergent" (i.e., more urgent) order pending.

The performances associated with the order flag can only be fully conceived when bound with other artefacts, its location, and people's movements. First, the flags are intended to call attention to *another artefact*—the order sheets. The flags are placed on the patient room doorframe right above a bin containing the actual order form, nurse flow sheets, and other documents that are part of the patient's

© Springer International Publishing Switzerland 2014
P. Bjørn, C. Østerlund, *Sociomaterial-Design*, Computer Supported Cooperative Work,
DOI 10.1007/978-3-319-12607-4_7

chart. Second, the *location* is essential. Much like the green X-ray folder in the Canadian ED used to alert nurses of patients returning from radiology, the flags are meant to act as beacons in the busy hallway, calling nurses' attention to a patient's room and, in particular, to the new orders given by a doctor. Third, the doctors introduced the flags because of a perceived problem of *mobility*—too much mobility. Doctors and nurses are constantly on the move, which makes it cumbersome to find people with whom one needs to communicate. The doctors have worked hard to introduce this seemingly simple information system in the hopes of freeing themselves from having to find nurses when giving an order. In other words, the doctors want to overcome the mobility concern by changing their interactions from a synchronous to an asynchronous interaction mediated by the flags and the order sheets.

The flags do not seem to have had the intended effect. Often red flags are displayed for a long time, seemingly without anybody taking notice. During the staff meeting, discussion first turns to whether it is reasonable to make the orders, and thus nurses' work, visible to everybody. Clara, an older nurse, describes how she missed a red flag the other day. The patient's family finally called it to her attention. "I felt awful!" Clara concludes. The other nurses all agree. The flags make them feel exposed by having pending work tasks made visible not only to colleagues, but also to patients' families (Fig. 7.1).

When the nurses raise their concerns, the flags' intra-actions with other artefacts, their location, and people's mobility also stand front and centre. The flag is

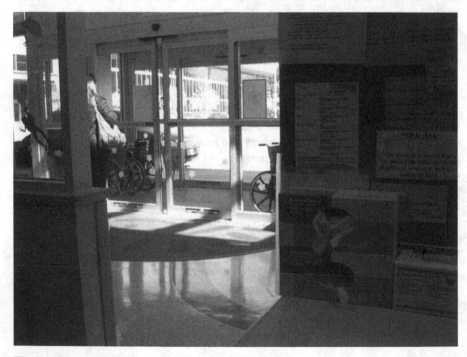

Fig. 7.1 Triage nurse view over the Emergency Department

not a pre-given artefact but part of larger and smaller engagements. To the nurses, however, these intra-actions are problematic. First, they have little interest in forging a bound among the order and the flags and thus having the flags mediate their communication with the doctors around orders. Sharon articulates a sentiment often heard among nurses: she worries that the flags will become "a substitute for communication." Nurses feel strongly that when doctors communicate an order with a flag, not through paper and face-to-face interaction, nurses lose the opportunity to question and give input on an order. In their daily work, nurses check the calculations of doctors' orders, suggest alternative possibilities, or simply want to know the rationale behind a particular order so as to be able to answer patients' or their families' questions. The flags bring them a step further away from care decisions.

Second, the nurses find the *location* of the flags problematic. By their conspicuous position mounted on the patient room doorframes, the flags inevitably include patients and their relatives as participants in this new artefact. The nurses are concerned about the patients' active involvement in the nurses' communication with doctors.

Third, the placement of the flags assumes that nurses *move* in and out of the patient exam rooms constantly, thus allowing them to see changes to the flags. Instead, they spend a significant amount of time at the heart of the ED in front of the whiteboard, coordinating and documenting their care. John, a senior physician, attempts to justify the new coordinative artefact. It is difficult, he argues, to find people, even doctors: "At night I give everybody [i.e., doctors] a phone. Then we can reach each other all the time and don't have to go hunting. I receive calls in the restroom." William, an ED doctor, suggests that the core problem is not that people cannot find each other but that the nurses should move around less. They should spend more time in the patients' rooms. William argues: "The nurses spend a lot of time in front of the whiteboard, while the docs run around like headless chickens." Clara points out that the residents (junior doctors) spend a considerable amount of time in the charting room. William insists: "Often it's impossible to find out when one nurse has taken over from another nurse. We need to get people back into the patient rooms where they belong, not sitting in front of the whiteboard or in the glass box [charting room]".

As in all other meetings, discussion of one artefact quickly leads to its physical properties and intra-actions with other artefacts, locations, and people's movements. First, Sharon suggests that they place the flags on the whiteboard. In other words, she suggests forging a bound between the new coordinative artefact and *other artefacts*, not only the orders but also the ED tracking whiteboard (Fig. 7.2).

The group discusses whether the whiteboard is already too cluttered. Jimmy, a secretary, brings up an idea, proposing that they allocate a slot for each team on the whiteboard where a magnetic flag would indicate pending orders. If they rotate the information on the board 90° they could make space for such fields. The suggestion is soon pushed aside by yet another idea from William, the doctor. He proposes placing all the orders in racks under the whiteboard. Each team should have its own order box. The senior physicians and the chart nurses can see if a team is getting behind on their orders or if there are any urgent orders pending, he explains. They

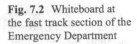

Fig. 7.2 Whiteboard at the fast track section of the Emergency Department

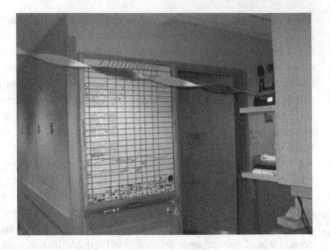

would not have to walk from door to door when rounding, William suggests, and he concludes by arguing that such a change would help nurses detect when colleagues need help.

In reaction to the argument, the ED staff starts imagining new bounding of the flags with other artefacts, locations, and mobility patterns. The new boundings would allow all doctors and nurses to monitor the number of pending orders for each team. Much like the yellow notes in the Canadian ED or the expect sheets in the U.S. ED, the number of order sheets compiled in a team's box would indicate pending work or, in other words, how much catching up nurses of a particular team would have to do. The physical properties associated with the flag and the whiteboard would need to be altered in order to create this bounding. Without such changes, the bounding would not be practical. The flags could be changed into coloured magnets. At the same time, it would require a reconfiguration of the content and format of the whiteboard, which may make it too cluttered. This solution would secure the intra-actions between the flag and the paper-based order sheet.

Second, in this new *location* the bounded flags and the orders would draw attention not only to one patient's room, but also to all patient rooms represented on the whiteboard. The flags would operate in a place associated with the management of work in the entire ED, and not solely the care for an individual patient.

Third, the new arrangements change the flags' intra-actions with the *movements* not only of doctors and nurses, but also of the patients and their significant others. No longer will the flags be under the gaze of relatives as they pace the hallways. More importantly, the changes bring the flags closer to where nurses and doctors spend significant amounts of time doing their paperwork—in front of the tracking whiteboard. Furthermore, the new intra-actions might alter how doctors and nurses move during rounds, as suggested by William. They would no longer have to walk from door to door; instead, they could stay in front of the whiteboard. Nurses could likewise monitor each other's workload from one location instead of moving around the ward.

Breaking bounds often leads to undesired consequences. As a response to William, Joyce tersely points out that bringing the orders to the whiteboard would further take the patient chart apart: "You need the order with the nursing flow sheet." William agrees. As it is, the chart already gets distributed all over the ED. The secretary manager and Jimmy nod their heads in agreement. They know the problem. They gather the charts daily when patients leave the ED, and then sort and send the assembled documents to the records department. At stake here is the bounding between the orders and the nursing flow sheet. Forging an entity out of the flags and orders comes at a price. It would break up the highly valued bound between the order sheet and the flow sheet, the latter being used at the patient's bedside. Neither doctors nor nurses seem willing to give up such an important artefact and the agential cut associated with it.

Joyce takes steps to end the meeting. She suggests that they should let the experiment with team A's flags go on for a bit longer. "It has not really been tested yet." She stresses that the flags should not be a substitute for communication among nurses and doctors. John adds his two cents: "The flags are just a substitute until the day we all have phones operated into our ears." Joyce closes the conversation by suggesting that they look into the possibility of adding "order boxes" under the whiteboard. With many issues raised and few resolved, the group leaves.

The reconfiguration of sociomaterial practices that follow the negotiations of new boundings often leads to conflicts. The ED staff's performances as doctors and nurses, respectively, ties directly into to the carefully woven artefacts, locations, and practices established and maintained during their meetings: Who is ultimately responsible for the order and who would get penalized if the communication breaks down? The nurses worry that by turning the communication about orders into an asynchronous interaction they would lose an important role in patient treatment—their ability to negotiate care regimens with doctors face-to-face before an order is set in stone. As doctors and nurses negotiate new and old boundings, they also debate the rules governing their responsibilities and power structures. Inevitably, conflicts emerge as new re-configures old. These are truly sociomaterial entanglements going beyond mere representational and epistemic considerations. The ED world is made and remade.

Part III
Sociomaterial-Design

Chapter 8
Boundaries and Intra-Actions

At first glance, any attempt to articulate a sociomaterial-design approach seems insurmountable, an oxymoron. Despite their shared commitment to a practice-based approach and the importance of materiality, they appear to turn their noses in opposite directions. One privileges the artefact while the other rejects any distinction between the human and the material. One does not question the boundaries associated with an artefact; the other insists no boundary is set in stone. One tends to look for inter-actions between the social and the technical; the other swears to intra-actions. Is it impossible to bring Ada and Alan together?

Barad (Barad 2007), with a little help from Haraway (Haraway 1994), offers us a way out of the conundrum. She insists on the importance of the boundaries and artefacts already constructed, but also the necessity of interrogating and refiguring them. In Barad's words:

> The intra-action involving the subject-object problematizes natural, pure, and innocent separations, but not in a way which reaches for the rapid dissolution of boundaries. Boundaries are not our enemies, they are necessary for making meaning, but this does not make them innocent. Boundaries have real material consequences—cuts are agentially positioned and accountability is mandatory. (Barad 1996, p. 187)

Boundaries are not our enemies as long as we question the boundaries for particular artefacts and refigure the boundaries in our analysis and design practices it is not a problem. We cannot approach boundaries as pre-existing. Yet, we face a world sliced and diced by agential cuts (Barad 2003), which means that we have to face the artefacts already out there and the distinctions and boundaries of which they are a part. As the previous examples have demonstrated, EDs are chock full of artefacts painfully configured and re-configured over generations and bound, but not shackled, to doctors' and nurses' current performances. By questioning and refiguring those prominent artefacts and their intra-actions additional agential cuts emerge along with new possibilities for design. Sociomaterial-design offers a few added degrees of freedom.

First, sociomaterial-design is about building sociomaterial artefacts, changing the conditions for the how technologies can be bound in practice. In contrast, approaches assuming a separation of the social and technical tend to get stuck in

© Springer International Publishing Switzerland 2014
P. Bjørn, C. Østerlund, *Sociomaterial-Design,* Computer Supported Cooperative Work,
DOI 10.1007/978-3-319-12607-4_8

epistemological concerns: What knowledge representations work best in one setting versus another? What epistemological sense-making practices should a system support? Sociomaterial design allows the researcher to take a step further and recognize that the sociomaterial practice we contribute to and the artefacts we come in contact with have real material and ontological consequences. The world on which we act is dynamic. Therefore, instead of designing for how the world immediately appears to us, we should look closer and may be new sociomaterial entanglements will unfold. Bohr's two experimental setups proved light to be a wave *and* a particle depending on how the artefacts were configured (Barad 1996). Likewise, sociomaterial-design has ontological consequences. When a nurse picks up a pile of expect sheets, she is dealing with a wave of patients on their way to the ED. If she slips out one expect sheet, she faces a singular patient hurling toward the ED. Likewise, when the Canadian ED transformed the paper-based triage template into a digital triage template, they did more than move a representational strategy from one artefact to another. They disconnected several sociomaterial practices that afterwards had to be re-entangled in new ways. Performing in the ED was no longer the same for the nurse; however, exactly how the conditions had changed was not very obvious.

8.1 Open-ended Artefacts

Sociomaterial-designers face open-ended artefacts. The physical material form of the artefact does not create the boundaries, but instead includes/excludes various dynamic sociomaterial practices at particular times. When healthcare professionals act in practice, they enact the artefacts in different ways. The artefacts are not stable entities, but instead dynamic entities that we can only approach by freezing a point in time to see what is revealed there. The artefact can be one yellow note in the Canadian ED or a [queue-of-yellow-notes]. It can be a [flow-sheet-in-a-rack-at-triage-nurses-moving-across-identifying-the-patient] or a [flow-sheet-at-registration-clerk-handling-patient-to-nurse]. When healthcare professionals enact an artefact, they bind together through inclusion while bracketing out what makes the boundaries for the artefact related to the purpose of the practice at a particular time. Each artefact bounds the world differently and performs distinct agential cuts. It gives us the freedom to play with how we, as well as practitioners, bound the world. For instance, sociomaterial-designers do not have to limit their design considerations to one type of material, such as desktops computers with ordinary keyboards and screens. Instead the sociomaterial-design approach encourages us to constantly think in terms of different and dynamic materials since, if we are to design for dynamic boundings of artefacts, it makes sense to think about dynamic material. One can come to use sociomaterial-design practices that demand the exploration of the larger and smaller entanglements in which all boundings and their artefacts exist. Just as the doctors and nurses in the U.S. ED mentioned in this book explored larger and smaller sociomaterial entanglements associated with a new order flag, so can sociomaterial-designers. Exploring open-ended boundaries can also help sociomaterial-designers understand how a new boundings will cause ripples through a sociomaterial entanglement. This exploration allows us to systematically explore the sociomaterial entanglement without reducing the complexity we know exists (Ciborra 1996).

8.2 Move Beyond Affordances and Constraints

In a sociomaterial-design approach it doesn't make sense to talk about specific affordances and constraints associated with particular types of artefacts. Affordances and constraints come with specific boundings and the boundaries they erect. Given that any artefact is part of larger and smaller entanglements, and thus boundings, shifting—and sometimes conflicting—affordances and constraints may be associated with the same artefact. This means that there is no direct causal link between the artefact and particular affordances and constraints. In the Canadian case of the new triage system, we cannot associate specific affordances and constraints with the digital artefact implemented, nor with the way the artefact interacted with the social setting. The real material consequences come with the boundings performed by the practitioners, and the digital artefact does not offer us many insights in and of itself. These involve the bounding of many artefacts, locations, and people's movements.

Sociomaterial-design is practice-oriented. Tracing boundings performed by practitioners offers important insights, but we must not lose sight of the design agenda and become lost in nitty-gritty details. Complex knowledge about sociomaterial performances can easily remain impractical for design researchers, whose interest is to create smart, simple design solutions. When we in the sociomaterial literature face terms like "assemblages" (Law 2004), "practice-order bundles" (Schatzki 2002), "mangle of practice" (Pickering 1995), and "entanglements" (Barad 2007), they easily resemble large Georgian knots, which we readily can whack at any empirical observation, but never pick apart. A sociomaterial-design approach allows us to leave the Georgian knot to the history books and instead trace the strings into the entanglement. As the U.S. and Canadian cases illustrate, we soon find carefully crafted boundings all nested in larger and smaller entanglements. We can trace these through sociomaterial practices, much like children play cat's cradle (Haraway 1994). Jacob's ladder leads us to the Eiffel Tower, on to cup and saucer, and finally cat's cradle. But, what strings do we trail, what boundings will assist us in creating sociomaterial-design solutions?

Examining our empirical data, we have created an analytical process that assists sociomaterial-designers in managing an otherwise overwhelming entanglement. We suggest that sociomaterial-designers take their point of departure from prominent artefacts that practitioners will readily identify. These offer a good point of departure as many boundings evolve around them. To identify the most important boundings for the sociomaterial-designer, we propose a three-step analytical process that brings the sociomaterial-designer from the artefact to the actual sociomaterial performances and intra-actions central to the organizational endeavor. First, we look for how practitioners bound multiple artefacts. Second, we articulate the bounding of these artefacts and their locations. Third, we set the analysis in motion and seek the bounding of artefacts, their locations, and people's movements. Returning to the cat's cradle metaphor, we first identify the strings in play, recognizing that what appears at first glance as a pre-given artefact may indeed be part of larger and smaller interwoven strings, some of which might be equally important to our investigation. Second, we explore the threads' locations extended between the hands of players, again acknowledging that these places are part of the boundings defining the game. Last but not least, we set the game in motion by following the way the strings change position as they move from hand to hand, from one participant to the next.

The three steps offer a structured way to enter the entanglement. It is a way for Ada and Alan to collaborate. The bounding of artefacts will likely reveal intra-actions easily overlooked by the designer (Ada), but easily detected by the ethnographer (Alan). It is significant that the new design of artefacts (e.g., digital designs and information system) take into account how the artefact is co-constitutive of the practice with other artefacts when deciding on how to re-configure the physical materiality including considerations and imaginations of what makes design material, for example, light, smell, sensors, or fabric. With the bounding of newfound artefacts and locations we articulate the field of action within which the boundings of the practitioners take place. An understanding of this field of action is essential for productive design, as the changing of location may bring forth unforeseen bounding practices. The sociomaterial-designer bounds the artefacts in their locations with people's movements. It allows the designer to truly explore the performances associated with specific boundings and their artefacts. As architects must study the flow of people through a building, so must the sociomaterial-designer take movement into account to fully understand how new designs will support or disrupt existing boundings and their performances.

We have now created the theoretical foundations for sociomaterial-design, and we have demonstrated how such an approach changes the focus when we study and design healthcare practices in EDs from an empirical perspective. We have suggested a three-step process through which Ada and Alan can engage and collaborate together when they are creating design interventions into the practices. Also, we have pointed to how the design of digital artefacts within the ED can be explored critically before making any important decisions as to which types of material properties the new design intervention must contain. However, at this stage it is important that we include the space to think about how sociomaterial-design would look in a different setting than healthcare. Healthcare practice is a special type of practice organized in particular ways, but what happens to sociomaterial-design if we move beyond the healthcare domain?

References

Barad, K.: Meeting the universe halfway: realism and social constructivism without contradiction. In: Nelson, L.H., Nelson, J. (eds.) Feminism, Science, and the Philosophy of Science, pp. 161–194. Kluwer, London (1996)

Barad, K.: Posthumanist performativity: toward an understanding of how matter comes to matter. Signs: J. Women Cult. Soc. **28**(3), 801–831 (2003)

Barad, K.: Meeting the Universe Halfway: Quantum Physics and the Entanglement of Matter and Meaning. Duke University Press, Durham (2007)

Ciborra, C.: The platform organiation: recombining strategies, structures, and surprises. Organ. Sci. **7**(2), 103–118 (1996)

Haraway, D.: A game of cat's cradle: science studies, feminist theory, cultural studies. Configurations **2**(1), 59–71 (1994)

Law, J.: After Methods: Mess in Social Science Research. Routledge, New York (2004)

Pickering, A.: The Mangle of Practice, Time, Agency and Science. University of Chicago Press, Chicago (1995)

Schatzki, T.R.: The Site of the Social: A Philosophical Account of the Constitution of Social Life and Change. Pennsylvania State University Press, University Park (2002)

Chapter 9
Sociomaterial-Design Beyond Healthcare

In this book, the domain of interest has been healthcare practice and, in particular, the work practices within EDs in North America. However healthcare practice is a particular type of practice, creating particular conditions for conducting sociomaterial-design. One of the basic conditions is that when you, as a sociomaterial-designer, enter the healthcare practice within a hospital, you encounter people, practices, and artefacts that all move around—making it possible for you to tag along. The actual practice of healthcare practitioners is very visible since interaction with a patient is a physical activity and the traditional coordination and organization of the work includes observable practices using tools such as clipboards, chart-racks, and whiteboards. Sociomaterial-design is not a restricted approach to only study healthcare; it is a general approach to the study of work practices with the aim of designing technology. However, sociomaterial-design will take different forms when executed within other domains. It is not within the scope of this book to completely unfold the meaning of sociomaterial-design in all different kinds of domains. However, it is in the scope of this book to consider and propose the questions that need to be addressed when conducting sociomaterial-design in settings other than healthcare practices. Thus, the questions we address in this chapter is how the conditions for conducting sociomaterial-design change or are transformed when introduced into domains different from healthcare, and what questions should the sociomaterial designer address when initiating such new investigations.

The first pertinent aspect of healthcare work is that it mostly consists of visually observable or tangible practices. Thus, the main question we as sociomaterial designers have to ask ourselves when moving out of healthcare is: How can we conduct sociomaterial-design in situations where the study of work is less tangible?

In our society, technology is an embedded part of the practices we engage with, and the introduction of technology changes the way work is organized and produced. Examples are to be found in studies of office work, such as Lucy Suchman's study of copy machines (Suchman 1987) or the excellent studies of control rooms (Harper et al. 1989; Heath and Luff 1992). These and others alike all point to how studying work in offices or in control rooms includes careful reflections on the participants' points of view when understanding the role of artefacts, and that introducing new technologies does impact work. However, what these studies were unable

© Springer International Publishing Switzerland 2014   97
P. Bjørn, C. Østerlund, *Sociomaterial-Design,* Computer Supported Cooperative Work,
DOI 10.1007/978-3-319-12607-4_9

to explore was how office work has become increasingly digitalized over the last several decades, meaning that people's movements and use of artefacts have transformed in a way that makes them less visible, tangible, and observable. Increasingly, internal mail systems are used less, and are instead being replaced by electronic systems (some by email, others by specialized designed systems like e-invoice). These shifts require us as researchers to engage with new approaches in terms of understanding the practices for the technology in use. Various researchers have developed approaches and analytical lenses directed at understanding technology in use practices outside healthcare; for example, "technology frames" (Orlikowski and Gash 1994; Bjørn et al. 2006), "genre repertoire" (Yates and Orlikowski 2002; Østerlund 2007), and "email overload" (Bellotti et al. 2005; Dabbish and Kraut 2006). However, each of these approaches does not take into account the sociomaterial practices that are included in such technology-in-use practices, but tend to take the perspective of focusing solely on the technology. There are multiple reasons that explain why earlier research on technology-in-use practices does not include the socialmaterial practices that serve as the foundation for the work under study. An important one is that, to understand the digitalized work practices that consist of how modern office work functions today, the sociomaterial-designer cannot shadow people and paper documents in the processes that occur. People do not interact in the same way with physical artefacts. Instead, much of the collaboration in modern office work takes place while the participants are located in front of their computer screens accessing multiple applications in multiple ways. In addition, there are several workplaces where collaborating across geography is the norm for work. For example, software development is now in most cases organized as collaboration across geographic borders, languages, and time spans (Bjørn et al. 2014). What this means for us as sociomaterial-designers is that understanding how participants are bounding artefacts in sociomaterial practices cannot be accomplished by applying the same observation techniques and tools as when observing hospital work. The crucial artefacts are simply not necessarily physical artefacts we can see move around. The question then becomes: Does the sociomaterial-design approach only function when observing physical labour, such as in hospitals or in factories? How can we identify the key artefacts if they are all digitally embedded within laptops, tablets, and smartphones? And if we manage to identify the key digital artefacts, how do we study how practitioners bound their artefacts when they work and collaborate? Do we need to modify the three types of bounding when we move into the global modern office?

We argue that it *is* possible to apply the sociomaterial-design approach also to modern office work in global collaborative setups heavily embedded within a diverse set of digital devices and infrastructures. However, it requires careful considerations into identifying what the crucial artefact might entail and how these are bounded in practice. When entering a large global organization with the purpose of studying global collaborative practices in a sociomaterial-design perspective it is clear that what we encounter immediately are the local work practices, and, as such, how the participants in the local organization move around, and many of the visible artefacts (such as printers, computers, and whiteboards) might give little indication for which artefacts are key for the global work and how we should take the bounding of these into account when designing.

If we start delving into a curiosity about how people in large global organization manage to collaborate despite the discontinuities in geography, time, and culture—and still want to maintain a sociomaterial interest—the starting point is to pursue a genuine interest in how global work is accomplished in practice. Observing global work as sociomaterial-designers, we become drawn to the observation of remote-technology-mediated meetings where geographically distributed participants collaborate. After all, at first glance global collaboration must be where people interact, and this would seem to be the meetings. We, as sociomaterial-designers studying global work, move with the participants into fancy video rooms and study how meetings are executed. Studying technology-mediated meetings (Mark et al. 2003), we might be surprised at how local artefacts such as Kanban boards (Matthiesen et al. 2014), war-room posters, and Post-it notes (Bjørn and Christensen 2011) are important artefacts that are part of organizing the collaboration. Introducing sociomaterial-design as an analytical lens to observe and unpack this setting suggests that an important bounding practice that should be investigated concerns *the bounding practices where artefacts are bounded in terms of their relations towards other physical locations at particular times.* An artefact such as a local Kanban board could be related to participants who are in remote locations during synchronous interaction through (e.g., video conferencing). However, while investigating such *boundings, it is critical that such relations tend to be only temporary connections and disappear with digital disconnect.* Likewise, the practices at different geographical locations could produce different boundings concerning the same artefact due to the differences in proximity to the artefact.

Interestingly, the majority of the collaborative work in a global setup actually happens outside of meetings, and as such we do not get access to observe this kind of work by observing video meetings. When we follow the participants back to their desks to observe their work, we suddenly find ourselves observing the back of, for instance, a software developer sitting in front of two large screens for many hours. At first, this might give the indication that the software developer works without any direct interaction with others and that the only artefact is the computer on the desk. However, if we start to look closer, we will see that the computer is not one artefact. Instead, the computer resembles the artefactual multiplicity we also find in healthcare (Bjørn and Hertzum 2011), and it brings together many collaborative applications in new constellations that are constantly changing and in close collaboration with others. The software developer might have an source-code environment open, several emails with different highlights, an Instant Messenger application, a blog, several documents from different documents repositories, and an electronic to-do list (Jensen and Bjørn 2012). All of these artefacts are crucial for the software developer to be able to do her work and collaborate with others, and if we as sociomaterial-designers want to understand the practices we need to focus on *how the participants bound together artefacts—not only physical artefacts, but also digital artefacts.* It might be that, to complete a particular activity, several digital artefacts together with a printed pile of paper is what makes the bounding of artefacts. Bounding multiple artefacts thus includes the bounding of particular instances of computer applications. It is not the computer application in itself which becomes bounded—it is the particular email, the particular source file, or the particular text file which becomes bounded together and meaningful for the participants. There is still much work to be done in understanding how multiple digital artefacts become bounded in the practices of global collaboration. One suggested approach is to think in terms of documentscape practices (Christensen and Bjørn 2014). Documentscape is a concept that describes the interlinked nature of various digital documents in global software development that together form the fundamental backbone of the document collaboration. The term also describes how the document collaboration changes and transforms over time. The relations within a documentscape are created through intertextuality, sequentiality, and autonomy of single documents, which together create a whole. From a sociomaterial-design perspective the documentscape is an interesting analytical device that depicts certain types of bounding of multiple digital artefacts. However, we as sociomaterial designers still need to do more work to determine and identify ways to address and think about digital bounding practices when engaging with modern office work.

In modern office work, if we are to investigate the bounding of people's movements and an artefact, we might at first only observe that the participant does not move very much—with the exception of going to and from meeting rooms. Does this mean that studying the bounding practices of people's movements is irrelevant in global office work? We would say no. People's movements are very important, however we need to think of the "movement" in a different way when studying global office work, since movements might not be detectable by simply walking between the print room, the meeting room, and the desk. Instead, movements might be in terms of devices. In modern global workspaces, people have various devices, such as laptops, desktops, tablets, smart phones, etc. When studying global work, the "movement" between devices is an important bounding to investigate. What kind of bounding practices do participants enact across instances of applications when they are collaborating globally on their smart phone, compared to their desktop or laptop? Such work risks blurring the distinction between life and work and thus the locations relevant for boundings, since participants are also available outside normal office hours and in locations other than the office. This means that participants bound what kind of interaction they can have on their smartphone, compared to the interaction they have on their laptop. It could be that some participants have installed different applications on different devices to help them create the boundaries. You could be able to check your email on your smartphone, but the kind of email interaction you have on the smartphone is different compared to the email interaction you have on the laptop because you bound the email application practices in different ways. Therefore, *understanding the bounding practices of people's movements and artefacts in modern office work must include investigations of how participants include or exclude digital devices in certain types of boundings, as well as where the location might be—being outside or inside the office.*

Finally, if we are to investigate modern global office work in a sociomaterial-design perspective, the bounding of location also changes. When global collaborators interact, their locations are not shared and as such we need to rethink how location and bounding practices might be more than the location of the artefact. If the single artefact is the application within different devices, the location of the artefact includes the location of the device. Devices move between pockets, bags, tables, and office spaces, as well as enter into other organizations or spaces such as the home. For each movement, the location of the artefact determined by the location of the application on the device will be bounded depending upon the work of the participant as well as the infrastructures available at the different locations. It might be that a software architect is visiting a client bringing a laptop, and she might have access to the Internet and thus the different source files that are important to demonstrate particular user interfaces for the client. Therefore, the location of the source file artefact becomes determined by the location of the laptop and whether or not the laptop has access to the Internet. *Investigating the sociomaterial practices in global work thus includes investigations of the bounding involved when participants work with artefacts, the location of these artefacts on devices, and the devices' access to infrastructures, which might or might not provide access to the artefacts.*

In this chapter, we have attempted to reflect on how to think about sociomaterial-design beyond the healthcare domain, and begin to point to what such investigations might entail. We do not claim to have identified the complete set of boundings that are important when moving outside of the healthcare domain, but what we have done is to provide some indications as to where sociomaterial designer should begin their journey. We are certain that there are many aspects we have not considered that are crucially important. Therefore, we encourage others to take up where we left off and consider what Sociomaterial-Design might mean to their domain of interest.

References

Bellotti, V., Ducheneaut, N., et al.: Quality versus quantity: email-centrix task management and its relation with overload. Hum. Comput. Interact. **20**, 89–138 (2005)

Bjørn, P., Christensen, L.R.: Relation work: creating socio-technical connections in global engineering. European Conference on Computer Supported Cooperative Work (ECSCW), pp. 133–152. Kluwer Academic, Aarhus (2011)

Bjørn, P., Hertzum, M.: Artefactual multiplicity: a study of emergency-department whiteboards. Comput. Support. Coop. Work (CSCW): Int. J. **20**(1), 93 (2011)

Bjørn, P., Scupola, A., et al.: Expanding technological frames towards mediated collaboration: groupware adoption in virtual learning teams. Scand. J. Inf. Syst. **18**(2), 3–42 (2006)

Bjørn, P., Bardram, J., et al.: Global software development in a CSCW perspective. Workshop paper for Computer Supported Cooperative Work and Social Computing (CSCW). ACM, Baltimore (2014)

Christensen, L., Bjørn, P.: Documentscape: intertextuallity, sequentiality and autonomy at work. ACM CHI Conference on Human Factors in Computing Systems, ACM, Toronto (2014)

Dabbish, L., Kraut, R.: Email overload at work: an analysis of facors associated with email strain. In: Proceedings of the 2006 ACM Conference on Computer Supported Cooperative Work, pp. 431–440, ACM, Banff (2006)

Harper, R., Hughes, J., et al.: Working in harmony: an examination of computer technology in air traffic control. European Conference on Computer Supported Cooperative Work, Gatwick (1989)

Heath, C., Luff, P.: Collaboration and control: crisis management and multimedia technology in London underground line control rooms. Comput. Support. Coop. Work (CSCW): Int. J. **1**, 69–94 (1992)

Jensen, R.E., Bjørn, P.: Divergence and convergence in global software development: cultural complexities as societal structures. In: COOP: Design of Cooperative Systems, pp. 123–136. Springer, France (2012)

Mark, G., Abrams, S., et al.: Group-to-group distance collaboration: examining the "Space Between". Proceedings of the Eighth European Conference on Computer Supported Cooperative Work, Helsinki, Finland, 14–18 Sept. 2003, pp. 99–118. Kluwer Academic, Netherlands (2003)

Matthiesen, S., Bjørn, P., et al.: Figure out how to code with the hands of others: recognizing cultural blind spots in global software development. Computer Supported Cooperative Work (CSCW). ACM, Baltimore (2014)

Orlikowski, W.J., Gash, D.C.: Technological frames: making sense of information technology in organizations. ACM Trans. Inf. Syst. **12**(2), 174–207 (1994)

Østerlund, C.: Genre combinations: a window into dynamic communication practices. J. Manage. Inform. Syst. **23**(4), 81–108 (2007)

Suchman, L.: Plans and Situated Actions. The Problem of Human Machine Communication. Cambridge University Press, Cambridge (1987)

Yates, J., Orlikowski, W.: Genre systems: structuring interaction through communicative norms. J. Bus. Commun. **39**(13), 13–35 (2002)

Chapter 10
Implications of Sociomaterial-Design

The sociomaterial-design agenda has implications for researchers and practitioners who are designing new coordinative artefacts for specific contexts, for example, when replacing paper-based systems with digital artefacts in a hospital setting, or collaborative systems for global work. We can no longer regard any of these artefacts as being pre-determined and stable. Instead, their boundaries are dynamic and created by the practitioners at different points in time, for particular purposes, through the bounding practices. People bound technologies in practice, and we should design with this in mind. Multiple boundings co-exist, each created by various practitioners for particular purposes. It is up to the sociomaterial-designer to identify relevant boundings by experimenting with and challenging the obvious boundaries that tend to appear to figure out whether other extremely relevant ways to bundle doings, materialities, and discourses co-exist and should be taken into account within new designs.

Our analysis suggests that the following key questions should be considered in such an experimental process. We propose that the answers to these questions must be carefully considered when deciding on new or revised designs of existing artefacts. The questions are:

1. What are the critical coordinative artefacts enacted in the sociomaterial practices under investigation?
2. For each critical artefact, what are the boundaries for particular people in particular situations? Subsequent questions to experiment with the boundaries are: What are the boundaries if the bounding concerns the intra-action between the artefact and other artefacts? What are the boundaries if the bounding process concerns the intra-actions between the artefact and various locations? What are the boundaries if the bounding process concerns the intra-actions between the artefact and people's movements?
3. For each bounding, what becomes present or absent for particular people at particular times?
4. What are the historical contexts and conflicting interests behind the different types of bounding for the artefact?

© Springer International Publishing Switzerland 2014
103
P. Bjørn, C. Østerlund, *Sociomaterial-Design,* Computer Supported Cooperative Work,
DOI 10.1007/978-3-319-12607-4_10

5. What new types of bounding will emerge for different types of new designs of artefacts, and which ones will disappear?

By integrating these questions into design, we might preserve essential sociomaterial practices in new design interventions, plus invent new sociomaterial practices based on new bundles of doings, materialities, and discourses. Sociomaterial-design strives to reduce the risk of accidentally cutting crucial strings in the ball of yarn when, for example, replacing paper-based coordinative practices with digital information systems.

We have explored how best to fuse a sociomaterial ontology with a design research agenda. This is quite a difficult journey, since we draw on two quite distinct and extensive literatures. On the one side, sociomateriality refuses the distinction between the social and the material and provides an analytical ontology for how practices are always bounded up and cannot be pulled apart easily (e.g. Pickering 1993; Orlikowski 2007; Mazmanian et al. 2014). On the other side, we have design (e.g. Bardram and Bossen 2005; Hertzum and Simonsen 2008; Simonsen and Robertsen 2013), which is characterized by an agenda of change and innovations through creating and reconfiguring design artefacts. So, our initial interest was to ask ourselves, what if we commit to understanding practice as sociomaterial complexities but still have an agenda to innovate and change the organization through information systems? What if we agree on the sociomaterial complexity of organizational practices, but do not simply want to stand passively by watching? What if we want to innovate and change organizational practice with the best intentions and without cutting essential relations? These are the questions that we have investigated in this book, and we put forward our sociomaterial-design approach as a way to answer these complex questions.

The hyphenated structure of sociomaterial-design underscores our interdisciplinary intentions, which not only bring a sociomaterial ontology to design, but also carry the design agenda to the sociomaterial project. We bind together the two to make a new entity. From the design agenda we take the interest in the designed IT-artefact as the centre of attention, but in contrast to other design science approaches, for example, sociotechnical approaches (Mumford 2006), we question the boundaries associated with a particular artefact as required by the sociomateriality agenda. Questioning the boundaries of artefact, sociomaterial-designers must trace how practitioners bound artefacts, locations, and their own movements in different ways. Untangling the numerous co-existing boundings is difficult and not straightforward. Nevertheless, we found that by examining the practices from three different perspectives and then fusing theses diverse angles we will arrive closer to the complexity of the sociomateriality of organizational practices, which can act as the starting point for innovation and design. The sociomaterial-designer starts by identifying artefacts prominent within practitioners' practices. With these in hand, the sociomaterial-designer maps important boundings by following a three-step process. First, the sociomaterial-designer traces larger and smaller entanglements by bounding artefacts into a new sociomaterial nexus of doings, materials, and discourses. These are likely to hint at boundings easily overlooked by the designer. Second, with artefact boundaries blurred, the sociomaterial-designer can now map the field of action within which the boundings take form. This is done by bounding and rebounding artefacts and locations, further articulating how specific performances rest on particular agential cuts. Finally, the sociomaterial-designer can highlight the dynamic aspect of important bounding artefacts of artefacts in their location, with the ways in which participants move to and from artefacts, in and out of locations. Over the course of the analytical process, the complexity of the practices arises and becomes the foundation for re-thinking the design of artefacts as well as an opening to think about designing the material properties with various different materialities. Our thinking should be free of concepts such as desktop, laptop, tablet, smartphone, and provide space for dynamic new materials (maybe soft, bendable, flexible, printable), which can be used to create new forms of artefacts with none-deterministic boundaries.

Our sociomaterial-design approach extends design research beyond epistemological concerns for knowledge representations into ontological and sociomaterial considerations. Also, we extend the literature on sociomateriality by providing rich empirical data from sociomaterial studies in a cross-case qualitative comparative analysis of organizational practices in healthcare, as well as by illustrating how sociomateriality can be directly relevant for current design research.

10.1 Final Remarks

This book has been a long journey of discussions, revisions, re-thinking, comparing, and critiquing. Not only has it been a journey forward in terms of writing and reading, it has also been a journey looking back and re-examining the large amount of rich empirical material we have and that is now part of who we are. When you have been closely involved in a practice over a long time, the experience becomes part of who you are as a researcher and it has been quite rewarding to go back, re-examine, and re-think these crucial practices that have so influenced our own research endeavours. As it is in all research, reflecting back on what you did, you will always seek to find a comprehensive narrative that makes the story of the past. However, it has been very worthwhile to challenge each other's narratives and critically examine both their differences and similarities.

We believe that the approach of sociomaterial-design is an important way forward in research, that can help to bring together researchers from the various disciplinary fields such as computer-supported cooperative work (CSCW), information systems (IS), human-computer interaction (HCI), design science (DS), participatory design (PD), and science and technology studies (STS), since we ourselves both travel across these disciplines with our research interests and believe we can fruitfully contribute to one another. The discussion on the basic nature of sociomaterial-design does not stop with this book, but instead is a continuous dynamic process through which hopefully other researchers will participate and engage with the debate. We see this book as a first step in a future process in which we manage to simultaneously pursue and embrace the complexity of practice, while also striving for simplicity in design.

References

Bardram, J., Bossen C.: A web of coordinative artefacts: collaborative work in a hospital ward. Group, Sanible Island, ACM (2005)

Hertzum, M., Simonsen J.: Positive effects of electronic patient records on three clinical activities. Int. J. Med. Inform. **77**(12), 809–817 (2008)

Mazmanian, M., Cohn, M., Dourish, P.: Dynamic reconfiguration in planetary exploration: a sociomaterial ethnography. MIS. Q. **38**(3), 831–848 (2014)

Mumford, E.: The story of socio-technical design: reflections on its successes, failures and potential. Inf. Syst. J. **16**, 317–342 (2006)

Orlikowski, W.: Sociomaterial practices: exploring technology at work. Org. Stud. **28**(9), 1435–1448 (2007)

Pickering, A.: The mangle of practice: agency and emergence in the sociology of science. Am. J. Sociol. **99**(3), 559–589 (1993)

Simonsen, J., Robertsen, T.: Participatory design: An introduction. International Handbook of Participatory Design, pp. 1–18. Routledge, London (2013)

Printed in the United States
By Bookmasters